F*cking Migraines

WELLNESS WARRIOR PRESS
www.wellnesswarriorpress.com

Copyright © 2020 by Wellness Warrior Press

ISBN: 978-1-990271-02-1

This journal belongs to...

_____

Summary

For each journal entry, return to this summary page and rate your overall pain / discomfort level
(1 being no pain and 10 being unbearable)

Entry #	Date	Rating	Notes / Suspected Triggers
1			
2			
3			
4			
5			
6			
7			
8			
9			
10			
11			
12			
13			
14			
15			
16			
17			
18			
19			
20			
21			
22			
23			
24			
25			
26			
27			
28			
29			
30			

Summary — continued

For each journal entry, return to this summary page and
rate your overall pain / discomfort level
(1 being no pain and 10 being unbearable)

Entry #	Date	Rating	Notes / Suspected Triggers
31			
32			
33			
34			
35			
36			
37			
38			
39			
40			
41			
42			
43			
44			
45			
46			
47			
48			
49			
50			
51			
52			
53			
54			
55			
56			
57			
58			
59			
60			

My Calendar

	January	February	March	April	May	June	July	August	September	October	November	December
1												
2												
3												
4												
5												
6												
7												
8												
9												
10												
11												
12												
13												
14												
15												
16												
17												
18												
19												
20												
21												
22												
23												
24												
25												
26												
27												
28												
29												
30												
31												

Calendar Legend

Create your own legend using colors or codes.

☐ _____

☐ _____

☐ _____

☐ _____

☐ _____

☐ _____

☐ _____

☐ _____

Additional Notes

_____

_____

_____

_____

_____

_____

_____

_____

_____

_____

_____

_____

_____

_____

_____

Date:_____

START:	END:	DURATION:

MIGRAINE	CLUSTER	SINUS	TMJ	TENSION

PAIN LEVEL

1	2	3	4	5	6	7	8	9	10

Not too bad.   *Well, I'm not enjoying this.*   *Holy shit, make it stop!*

DETAILED DESCRIPTION

☐ Constant   ☐ Squeezing   ☐ Throbbing   ☐ Pounding
☐ Dull aching   ☐ Burning   ☐ Sharp   ☐ Debilitating

Other:_____

ONSET

☐ Slow   ☐ Average   ☐ Rapid   ☐ Sudden

WHERE DOES IT HURT, EXACTLY?

OTHER SYMPTOMS

☐ Lightheaded   ☐ Dizziness   ☐ Confusion
☐ Light sensitivity   ☐ Sound sensitivity   ☐ Auras
☐ Muscle stiffness   ☐ Muscle burning   ☐ Muscle aches

HOW ARE YOU FEELING OVERALL?

Feeling sick?

Mood	① ② ③ ④ ⑤ ⑥ ⑦ ⑧ ⑨ ⑩	☐ Nope!
Energy levels	① ② ③ ④ ⑤ ⑥ ⑦ ⑧ ⑨ ⑩	☐ Yes...
Mental clarity	① ② ③ ④ ⑤ ⑥ ⑦ ⑧ ⑨ ⑩	

☐ Nausea   ☐ Diarrhea   ☐ Vomiting   ☐ Sore throat
☐ Congestion   ☐ Coughing   ☐ Chills   ☐ Fever

Other symptoms: _____

LAST NIGHT'S SLEEP

Hours of Sleep: _____   Sleep Quality: ① ② ③ ④ ⑤

WEATHER

☐ Hot   ☐ Mild   ☐ Cold   BM Pressure: _____

☐ Dry   ☐ Humid   ☐ Wet   Allergen Levels: _____

☐ Sunny   ☐ Cloudy

STRESS LEVELS

None	Low	Medium	High	Max	@$#%!

FOOD / DRINKS + NON-RELIEF MEDICATION / SUPPLEMENTS

item / meal	time	meds / supplements	dose	time

How many drinks?

water   ① ② ③ ④ ⑤ ⑥ ⑦ ⑧ ⑨ ⑩

caffeine ① ② ③ ④ ⑤ ⑥ ⑦ ⑧ ⑨ ⑩

alcohol ① ② ③ ④ ⑤ ⑥ ⑦ ⑧ ⑨ ⑩

HORMONES

☐ Menstruating   ☐ Menopause   ☐ PMS   ☐ N/A | other

COMPUTER USE / READING

☐ None   ☐ Some   ☐ A lot   Total time: [____]

☐ Sitting   ☐ Standing ☐ Mixture   Breaks every: [____]

PHYSICAL ACTIVITY

☐ None   ☐ Minimal   ☐ Some   ☐ Sweatin'   ☐ I'm beat

DETAILS: _____

RELIEF MEASURES

☐ Medication   ☐ Massage   ☐ Sleep   ☐ Exercise

☐ Water   ☐ Cold/Ice   ☐ Heat/Bath   ☐ Other

DETAILS: _____

DID IT WORK?   ☐ Nope   ☐ A bit   ☐ Mostly   ☐ 100%

Notes

Date:_____

START: [ ]   **END:** [ ]   **DURATION:** [ ]

| MIGRAINE | CLUSTER | SINUS | TMJ | TENSION |

PAIN LEVEL

| 1 | 2 | 3 | 4 | 5 | 6 | 7 | 8 | 9 | 10 |

Not too bad.   *Well, I'm not enjoying this.*   *Holy shit, make it stop!*

DETAILED DESCRIPTION

☐ Constant   ☐ Squeezing   ☐ Throbbing   ☐ Pounding
☐ Dull aching   ☐ Burning   ☐ Sharp   ☐ Debilitating

Other:_____

ONSET

☐ Slow   ☐ Average   ☐ Rapid   ☐ Sudden

WHERE DOES IT HURT, EXACTLY?

OTHER SYMPTOMS

☐ Lightheaded   ☐ Dizziness   ☐ Confusion
☐ Light sensitivity   ☐ Sound sensitivity   ☐ Auras
☐ Muscle stiffness   ☐ Muscle burning   ☐ Muscle aches

HOW ARE YOU FEELING OVERALL?

Feeling sick?

Mood ① ② ③ ④ ⑤ ⑥ ⑦ ⑧ ⑨ ⑩   ☐ Nope!
Energy levels ① ② ③ ④ ⑤ ⑥ ⑦ ⑧ ⑨ ⑩   ☐ Yes...
Mental clarity ① ② ③ ④ ⑤ ⑥ ⑦ ⑧ ⑨ ⑩

☐ Nausea   ☐ Diarrhea   ☐ Vomiting   ☐ Sore throat
☐ Congestion   ☐ Coughing   ☐ Chills   ☐ Fever

Other symptoms: _____

LAST NIGHT'S SLEEP

Hours of Sleep: _____   Sleep Quality: ① ② ③ ④ ⑤

WEATHER

☐ Hot   ☐ Mild   ☐ Cold   BM Pressure: _____

☐ Dry   ☐ Humid   ☐ Wet   Allergen Levels: _____

☐ Sunny   ☐ Cloudy

STRESS LEVELS

| None | Low | Medium | High | Max | @$#%! |

FOOD / DRINKS + NON-RELIEF MEDICATION / SUPPLEMENTS

item / meal	time	meds / supplements	dose	time

How many drinks?

water ① ② ③ ④ ⑤ ⑥ ⑦ ⑧ ⑨ ⑩

caffeine ① ② ③ ④ ⑤ ⑥ ⑦ ⑧ ⑨ ⑩

alcohol ① ② ③ ④ ⑤ ⑥ ⑦ ⑧ ⑨ ⑩

HORMONES

☐ Menstruating   ☐ Menopause   ☐ PMS   ☐ N/A | other

COMPUTER USE / READING

☐ None   ☐ Some   ☐ A lot   Total time: [   ]

☐ Sitting   ☐ Standing   ☐ Mixture   Breaks every: [   ]

PHYSICAL ACTIVITY

☐ None   ☐ Minimal   ☐ Some   ☐ Sweatin'   ☐ I'm beat

DETAILS: _____

RELIEF MEASURES

☐ Medication ☐ Massage   ☐ Sleep   ☐ Exercise

☐ Water   ☐ Cold/Ice   ☐ Heat/Bath   ☐ Other

DETAILS: _____

DID IT WORK?   ☐ Nope   ☐ A bit   ☐ Mostly   ☐ 100%

Notes

Date:_____

START:	END:	DURATION:

MIGRAINE	CLUSTER	SINUS	TMJ	TENSION

PAIN LEVEL

1	2	3	4	5	6	7	8	9	10

Not too bad.   *Well, I'm not enjoying this.*   *Holy shit, make it stop!*

DETAILED DESCRIPTION

☐ Constant   ☐ Squeezing   ☐ Throbbing   ☐ Pounding
☐ Dull aching   ☐ Burning   ☐ Sharp   ☐ Debilitating

Other:_____

ONSET

☐ Slow   ☐ Average   ☐ Rapid   ☐ Sudden

WHERE DOES IT HURT, EXACTLY?

OTHER SYMPTOMS

☐ Lightheaded   ☐ Dizziness   ☐ Confusion
☐ Light sensitivity   ☐ Sound sensitivity   ☐ Auras
☐ Muscle stiffness   ☐ Muscle burning   ☐ Muscle aches

HOW ARE YOU FEELING OVERALL?

Feeling sick?

Mood ① ② ③ ④ ⑤ ⑥ ⑦ ⑧ ⑨ ⑩   ☐ Nope!

Energy levels ① ② ③ ④ ⑤ ⑥ ⑦ ⑧ ⑨ ⑩   ☐ Yes...

Mental clarity ① ② ③ ④ ⑤ ⑥ ⑦ ⑧ ⑨ ⑩

☐ Nausea   ☐ Diarrhea   ☐ Vomiting   ☐ Sore throat
☐ Congestion   ☐ Coughing   ☐ Chills   ☐ Fever

Other symptoms: _____

LAST NIGHT'S SLEEP

Hours of Sleep: _____   Sleep Quality: ① ② ③ ④ ⑤

WEATHER

☐ Hot   ☐ Mild   ☐ Cold   BM Pressure: _____

☐ Dry   ☐ Humid   ☐ Wet   Allergen Levels: _____

☐ Sunny   ☐ Cloudy

STRESS LEVELS

None	Low	Medium	High	Max	@$#%!

FOOD / DRINKS + NON-RELIEF MEDICATION / SUPPLEMENTS

item / meal	time	meds / supplements	dose	time

How many drinks?

water	① ② ③ ④ ⑤ ⑥ ⑦ ⑧ ⑨ ⑩
caffeine	① ② ③ ④ ⑤ ⑥ ⑦ ⑧ ⑨ ⑩
alcohol	① ② ③ ④ ⑤ ⑥ ⑦ ⑧ ⑨ ⑩

HORMONES

☐ Menstruating   ☐ Menopause   ☐ PMS   ☐ N/A | other

COMPUTER USE / READING

☐ None   ☐ Some   ☐ A lot   Total time: [   ]

☐ Sitting   ☐ Standing   ☐ Mixture   Breaks every: [   ]

PHYSICAL ACTIVITY

☐ None   ☐ Minimal   ☐ Some   ☐ Sweatin'   ☐ I'm beat

DETAILS: _____

RELIEF MEASURES

☐ Medication   ☐ Massage   ☐ Sleep   ☐ Exercise

☐ Water   ☐ Cold/Ice   ☐ Heat/Bath ☐ Other

DETAILS: _____

DID IT WORK?   ☐ Nope   ☐ A bit   ☐ Mostly   ☐ 100%

Notes

Date:_____

START:	END:	DURATION:

MIGRAINE	CLUSTER	SINUS	TMJ	TENSION

PAIN LEVEL

1	2	3	4	5	6	7	8	9	10

Not too bad.   *Well, I'm not enjoying this.*   *Holy shit, make it stop!*

DETAILED DESCRIPTION

☐ Constant   ☐ Squeezing   ☐ Throbbing   ☐ Pounding
☐ Dull aching   ☐ Burning   ☐ Sharp   ☐ Debilitating

Other:_____

ONSET

☐ Slow   ☐ Average   ☐ Rapid   ☐ Sudden

WHERE DOES IT HURT, EXACTLY?

OTHER SYMPTOMS

☐ Lightheaded   ☐ Dizziness   ☐ Confusion
☐ Light sensitivity ☐ Sound sensitivity ☐ Auras
☐ Muscle stiffness ☐ Muscle burning   ☐ Muscle aches

HOW ARE YOU FEELING OVERALL?

Feeling sick?

Mood	① ② ③ ④ ⑤ ⑥ ⑦ ⑧ ⑨ ⑩	☐ Nope!
Energy levels	① ② ③ ④ ⑤ ⑥ ⑦ ⑧ ⑨ ⑩	☐ Yes...
Mental clarity	① ② ③ ④ ⑤ ⑥ ⑦ ⑧ ⑨ ⑩	

☐ Nausea   ☐ Diarrhea   ☐ Vomiting   ☐ Sore throat
☐ Congestion   ☐ Coughing   ☐ Chills   ☐ Fever

Other symptoms: _____

LAST NIGHT'S SLEEP

Hours of Sleep: _____   Sleep Quality: ① ② ③ ④ ⑤

WEATHER

☐ Hot   ☐ Mild   ☐ Cold   BM Pressure: _____

☐ Dry   ☐ Humid   ☐ Wet   Allergen Levels: _____

☐ Sunny   ☐ Cloudy

STRESS LEVELS

None	Low	Medium	High	Max	@$#%!

FOOD / DRINKS + NON-RELIEF MEDICATION / SUPPLEMENTS

item / meal	time	meds / supplements	dose	time

How many drinks?

water   ① ② ③ ④ ⑤ ⑥ ⑦ ⑧ ⑨ ⑩
caffeine ① ② ③ ④ ⑤ ⑥ ⑦ ⑧ ⑨ ⑩
alcohol ① ② ③ ④ ⑤ ⑥ ⑦ ⑧ ⑨ ⑩

HORMONES

☐ Menstruating   ☐ Menopause   ☐ PMS   ☐ N/A | other

COMPUTER USE / READING

☐ None   ☐ Some   ☐ A lot   Total time: _____

☐ Sitting   ☐ Standing   ☐ Mixture   Breaks every: _____

PHYSICAL ACTIVITY

☐ None   ☐ Minimal   ☐ Some   ☐ Sweatin'   ☐ I'm beat

DETAILS: _____

RELIEF MEASURES

☐ Medication   ☐ Massage   ☐ Sleep   ☐ Exercise

☐ Water   ☐ Cold/Ice   ☐ Heat/Bath   ☐ Other

DETAILS: _____

DID IT WORK?   ☐ Nope   ☐ A bit   ☐ Mostly   ☐ 100%

Notes

Date:_____

START:	END:	DURATION:

MIGRAINE	CLUSTER	SINUS	TMJ	TENSION

PAIN LEVEL

1	2	3	4	5	6	7	8	9	10

Not too bad.   *Well, I'm not enjoying this.*   *Holy shit, make it stop!*

DETAILED DESCRIPTION

☐ Constant   ☐ Squeezing   ☐ Throbbing   ☐ Pounding
☐ Dull aching   ☐ Burning   ☐ Sharp   ☐ Debilitating

Other:_____

ONSET

☐ Slow   ☐ Average   ☐ Rapid   ☐ Sudden

WHERE DOES IT HURT, EXACTLY?

OTHER SYMPTOMS

☐ Lightheaded   ☐ Dizziness   ☐ Confusion
☐ Light sensitivity   ☐ Sound sensitivity   ☐ Auras
☐ Muscle stiffness   ☐ Muscle burning   ☐ Muscle aches

HOW ARE YOU FEELING OVERALL?   Feeling sick?

Mood	① ② ③ ④ ⑤ ⑥ ⑦ ⑧ ⑨ ⑩	☐ Nope!
Energy levels	① ② ③ ④ ⑤ ⑥ ⑦ ⑧ ⑨ ⑩	☐ Yes...
Mental clarity	① ② ③ ④ ⑤ ⑥ ⑦ ⑧ ⑨ ⑩	

☐ Nausea   ☐ Diarrhea   ☐ Vomiting   ☐ Sore throat
☐ Congestion   ☐ Coughing   ☐ Chills   ☐ Fever

Other symptoms: _____

LAST NIGHT'S SLEEP

Hours of Sleep: _____   Sleep Quality: ① ② ③ ④ ⑤

WEATHER

☐ Hot   ☐ Mild   ☐ Cold   BM Pressure: _____

☐ Dry   ☐ Humid   ☐ Wet   Allergen Levels: _____

☐ Sunny   ☐ Cloudy

STRESS LEVELS

None	Low	Medium	High	Max	@$#%!

FOOD / DRINKS + NON-RELIEF MEDICATION / SUPPLEMENTS

item / meal	time	meds / supplements	dose	time

How many drinks?

water   ① ② ③ ④ ⑤ ⑥ ⑦ ⑧ ⑨ ⑩

caffeine ① ② ③ ④ ⑤ ⑥ ⑦ ⑧ ⑨ ⑩

alcohol ① ② ③ ④ ⑤ ⑥ ⑦ ⑧ ⑨ ⑩

HORMONES

☐ Menstruating   ☐ Menopause   ☐ PMS   ☐ N/A | other

COMPUTER USE / READING

☐ None   ☐ Some   ☐ A lot   Total time: [   ]

☐ Sitting   ☐ Standing   ☐ Mixture   Breaks every: [   ]

PHYSICAL ACTIVITY

☐ None   ☐ Minimal   ☐ Some   ☐ Sweatin'   ☐ I'm beat

DETAILS: _____

RELIEF MEASURES

☐ Medication   ☐ Massage   ☐ Sleep   ☐ Exercise

☐ Water   ☐ Cold/Ice   ☐ Heat/Bath   ☐ Other

DETAILS: _____

DID IT WORK?   ☐ Nope   ☐ A bit   ☐ Mostly   ☐ 100%

Notes

Date:_____

START:	END:	DURATION:

| MIGRAINE | CLUSTER | SINUS | TMJ | TENSION |

PAIN LEVEL

1	2	3	4	5	6	7	8	9	10

Not too bad.   *Well, I'm not enjoying this.*   *Holy shit, make it stop!*

DETAILED DESCRIPTION

☐ Constant   ☐ Squeezing   ☐ Throbbing   ☐ Pounding
☐ Dull aching   ☐ Burning   ☐ Sharp   ☐ Debilitating

Other:_____

ONSET

☐ Slow   ☐ Average   ☐ Rapid   ☐ Sudden

WHERE DOES IT HURT, EXACTLY?

OTHER SYMPTOMS

☐ Lightheaded   ☐ Dizziness   ☐ Confusion
☐ Light sensitivity ☐ Sound sensitivity ☐ Auras
☐ Muscle stiffness ☐ Muscle burning   ☐ Muscle aches

HOW ARE YOU FEELING OVERALL?

Feeling sick?

Mood	① ② ③ ④ ⑤ ⑥ ⑦ ⑧ ⑨ ⑩	☐ Nope!
Energy levels	① ② ③ ④ ⑤ ⑥ ⑦ ⑧ ⑨ ⑩	☐ Yes...
Mental clarity	① ② ③ ④ ⑤ ⑥ ⑦ ⑧ ⑨ ⑩	

☐ Nausea   ☐ Diarrhea   ☐ Vomiting   ☐ Sore throat
☐ Congestion   ☐ Coughing   ☐ Chills   ☐ Fever

Other symptoms: _____

LAST NIGHT'S SLEEP

Hours of Sleep: _____   Sleep Quality: ① ② ③ ④ ⑤

WEATHER

☐ Hot   ☐ Mild   ☐ Cold   BM Pressure: _____

☐ Dry   ☐ Humid   ☐ Wet   Allergen Levels: _____

☐ Sunny   ☐ Cloudy

STRESS LEVELS

None	Low	Medium	High	Max	@$#%!

FOOD / DRINKS + NON-RELIEF MEDICATION / SUPPLEMENTS

item / meal	time	meds / supplements	dose	time

How many drinks?

water   ➪ ① ② ③ ④ ⑤ ⑥ ⑦ ⑧ ⑨ ⑩

caffeine ➪ ① ② ③ ④ ⑤ ⑥ ⑦ ⑧ ⑨ ⑩

alcohol ➪ ① ② ③ ④ ⑤ ⑥ ⑦ ⑧ ⑨ ⑩

HORMONES

☐ Menstruating   ☐ Menopause   ☐ PMS   ☐ N/A | other

COMPUTER USE / READING

☐ None   ☐ Some   ☐ A lot   Total time: [   ]

☐ Sitting   ☐ Standing   ☐ Mixture   Breaks every: [   ]

PHYSICAL ACTIVITY

☐ None   ☐ Minimal   ☐ Some   ☐ Sweatin'   ☐ I'm beat

DETAILS: _____

RELIEF MEASURES

☐ Medication   ☐ Massage   ☐ Sleep   ☐ Exercise

☐ Water   ☐ Cold/Ice   ☐ Heat/Bath   ☐ Other

DETAILS: _____

DID IT WORK?   ☐ Nope   ☐ A bit   ☐ Mostly   ☐ 100%

Notes

Date:_____

START: [ ] END: [ ] DURATION: [ ]

| MIGRAINE | CLUSTER | SINUS | TMJ | TENSION |

PAIN LEVEL

1	2	3	4	5	6	7	8	9	10

Not too bad.   *Well, I'm not enjoying this.*   *Holy shit, make it stop!*

DETAILED DESCRIPTION

☐ Constant   ☐ Squeezing   ☐ Throbbing   ☐ Pounding
☐ Dull aching   ☐ Burning   ☐ Sharp   ☐ Debilitating

Other:_____

ONSET

☐ Slow   ☐ Average   ☐ Rapid   ☐ Sudden

WHERE DOES IT HURT, EXACTLY?

OTHER SYMPTOMS

☐ Lightheaded   ☐ Dizziness   ☐ Confusion
☐ Light sensitivity   ☐ Sound sensitivity   ☐ Auras
☐ Muscle stiffness   ☐ Muscle burning   ☐ Muscle aches

HOW ARE YOU FEELING OVERALL?

Feeling sick?

Mood   ① ② ③ ④ ⑤ ⑥ ⑦ ⑧ ⑨ ⑩   ☐ Nope!

Energy levels   ① ② ③ ④ ⑤ ⑥ ⑦ ⑧ ⑨ ⑩   ☐ Yes...

Mental clarity   ① ② ③ ④ ⑤ ⑥ ⑦ ⑧ ⑨ ⑩

☐ Nausea   ☐ Diarrhea   ☐ Vomiting   ☐ Sore throat
☐ Congestion   ☐ Coughing   ☐ Chills   ☐ Fever

Other symptoms: _____

LAST NIGHT'S SLEEP

Hours of Sleep: _____   Sleep Quality: ① ② ③ ④ ⑤

WEATHER

☐ Hot   ☐ Mild   ☐ Cold   BM Pressure: _____

☐ Dry   ☐ Humid   ☐ Wet   Allergen Levels: _____

☐ Sunny   ☐ Cloudy

STRESS LEVELS

None	Low	Medium	High	Max	@$#%!

FOOD / DRINKS + NON-RELIEF MEDICATION / SUPPLEMENTS

item / meal	time	meds / supplements	dose	time

How many drinks?

water   ① ② ③ ④ ⑤ ⑥ ⑦ ⑧ ⑨ ⑩

caffeine ① ② ③ ④ ⑤ ⑥ ⑦ ⑧ ⑨ ⑩

alcohol ① ② ③ ④ ⑤ ⑥ ⑦ ⑧ ⑨ ⑩

HORMONES

☐ Menstruating   ☐ Menopause   ☐ PMS   ☐ N/A | other

COMPUTER USE / READING

☐ None   ☐ Some   ☐ A lot   Total time: [   ]

☐ Sitting   ☐ Standing   ☐ Mixture   Breaks every: [   ]

PHYSICAL ACTIVITY

☐ None   ☐ Minimal   ☐ Some   ☐ Sweatin'   ☐ I'm beat

DETAILS: _____

RELIEF MEASURES

☐ Medication   ☐ Massage   ☐ Sleep   ☐ Exercise

☐ Water   ☐ Cold/Ice   ☐ Heat/Bath   ☐ Other

DETAILS: _____

DID IT WORK?   ☐ Nope   ☐ A bit   ☐ Mostly   ☐ 100%

Notes

Date:_____

START:	END:	DURATION:

MIGRAINE	CLUSTER	SINUS	TMJ	TENSION

PAIN LEVEL

1	2	3	4	5	6	7	8	9	10

Not too bad.   *Well, I'm not enjoying this.*   *Holy shit, make it stop!*

DETAILED DESCRIPTION

☐ Constant ☐ Squeezing ☐ Throbbing ☐ Pounding
☐ Dull aching ☐ Burning ☐ Sharp ☐ Debilitating

Other:_____

ONSET

☐ Slow ☐ Average ☐ Rapid ☐ Sudden

WHERE DOES IT HURT, EXACTLY?

OTHER SYMPTOMS

☐ Lightheaded ☐ Dizziness ☐ Confusion
☐ Light sensitivity ☐ Sound sensitivity ☐ Auras
☐ Muscle stiffness ☐ Muscle burning ☐ Muscle aches

HOW ARE YOU FEELING OVERALL?   Feeling sick?

Mood	① ② ③ ④ ⑤ ⑥ ⑦ ⑧ ⑨ ⑩	☐ Nope!
Energy levels	① ② ③ ④ ⑤ ⑥ ⑦ ⑧ ⑨ ⑩	☐ Yes...
Mental clarity	① ② ③ ④ ⑤ ⑥ ⑦ ⑧ ⑨ ⑩	

☐ Nausea ☐ Diarrhea ☐ Vomiting ☐ Sore throat
☐ Congestion ☐ Coughing ☐ Chills ☐ Fever

Other symptoms: _____

LAST NIGHT'S SLEEP

Hours of Sleep: _____   Sleep Quality: ① ② ③ ④ ⑤

WEATHER

☐ Hot   ☐ Mild   ☐ Cold   BM Pressure: _____
☐ Dry   ☐ Humid   ☐ Wet   Allergen Levels: _____
☐ Sunny   ☐ Cloudy

STRESS LEVELS

None	Low	Medium	High	Max	@$#%!

FOOD / DRINKS + NON-RELIEF MEDICATION / SUPPLEMENTS

item / meal	time	meds / supplements	dose	time
		How many drinks?		

water ⟹ ① ② ③ ④ ⑤ ⑥ ⑦ ⑧ ⑨ ⑩
caffeine ⟹ ① ② ③ ④ ⑤ ⑥ ⑦ ⑧ ⑨ ⑩
alcohol ⟹ ① ② ③ ④ ⑤ ⑥ ⑦ ⑧ ⑨ ⑩

HORMONES

☐ Menstruating   ☐ Menopause   ☐ PMS   ☐ N/A | other

COMPUTER USE / READING

☐ None   ☐ Some   ☐ A lot   Total time: [____]
☐ Sitting   ☐ Standing   ☐ Mixture   Breaks every: [____]

PHYSICAL ACTIVITY

☐ None   ☐ Minimal   ☐ Some   ☐ Sweatin'   ☐ I'm beat
DETAILS: _____

RELIEF MEASURES

☐ Medication   ☐ Massage   ☐ Sleep   ☐ Exercise
☐ Water   ☐ Cold/Ice   ☐ Heat/Bath   ☐ Other
DETAILS: _____

DID IT WORK?   ☐ Nope   ☐ A bit   ☐ Mostly   ☐ 100%

Notes

Date:_____

START:	END:	DURATION:

MIGRAINE	CLUSTER	SINUS	TMJ	TENSION

PAIN LEVEL

1	2	3	4	5	6	7	8	9	10

Not too bad.　　　*Well, I'm not enjoying this.*　　　*Holy shit, make it stop!*

DETAILED DESCRIPTION

☐ Constant　　☐ Squeezing　　☐ Throbbing　　☐ Pounding
☐ Dull aching　☐ Burning　　　☐ Sharp　　　☐ Debilitating

Other:_____

ONSET

☐ Slow　　　☐ Average　　☐ Rapid　　☐ Sudden

WHERE DOES IT HURT, EXACTLY?

OTHER SYMPTOMS

☐ Lightheaded　　　☐ Dizziness　　　☐ Confusion
☐ Light sensitivity　☐ Sound sensitivity　☐ Auras
☐ Muscle stiffness　☐ Muscle burning　☐ Muscle aches

HOW ARE YOU FEELING OVERALL?

Feeling sick?

Mood	① ② ③ ④ ⑤ ⑥ ⑦ ⑧ ⑨ ⑩	☐ Nope!
Energy levels	① ② ③ ④ ⑤ ⑥ ⑦ ⑧ ⑨ ⑩	☐ Yes...
Mental clarity	① ② ③ ④ ⑤ ⑥ ⑦ ⑧ ⑨ ⑩	

☐ Nausea　　　☐ Diarrhea　　☐ Vomiting　　☐ Sore throat
☐ Congestion　☐ Coughing　　☐ Chills　　　☐ Fever

Other symptoms:_____

LAST NIGHT'S SLEEP

Hours of Sleep: _____   Sleep Quality: ① ② ③ ④ ⑤

WEATHER

☐ Hot   ☐ Mild   ☐ Cold   BM Pressure: _____

☐ Dry   ☐ Humid   ☐ Wet   Allergen Levels: _____

☐ Sunny   ☐ Cloudy

STRESS LEVELS

None	Low	Medium	High	Max	@$#%!

FOOD / DRINKS + NON-RELIEF MEDICATION / SUPPLEMENTS

item / meal	time	meds / supplements	dose	time

How many drinks?

water   → ① ② ③ ④ ⑤ ⑥ ⑦ ⑧ ⑨ ⑩

caffeine → ① ② ③ ④ ⑤ ⑥ ⑦ ⑧ ⑨ ⑩

alcohol → ① ② ③ ④ ⑤ ⑥ ⑦ ⑧ ⑨ ⑩

HORMONES

☐ Menstruating   ☐ Menopause   ☐ PMS   ☐ N/A | other

COMPUTER USE / READING

☐ None   ☐ Some   ☐ A lot   Total time: [   ]

☐ Sitting   ☐ Standing   ☐ Mixture   Breaks every: [   ]

PHYSICAL ACTIVITY

☐ None   ☐ Minimal   ☐ Some   ☐ Sweatin'   ☐ I'm beat

DETAILS: _____

RELIEF MEASURES

☐ Medication   ☐ Massage   ☐ Sleep   ☐ Exercise

☐ Water   ☐ Cold/Ice   ☐ Heat/Bath   ☐ Other

DETAILS: _____

DID IT WORK?   ☐ Nope   ☐ A bit   ☐ Mostly   ☐ 100%

Notes

Date:_____

START:	END:	DURATION:

| MIGRAINE | CLUSTER | SINUS | TMJ | TENSION |

PAIN LEVEL

1	2	3	4	5	6	7	8	9	10

Not too bad.   *Well, I'm not enjoying this.*   *Holy shit, make it stop!*

DETAILED DESCRIPTION

☐ Constant   ☐ Squeezing   ☐ Throbbing   ☐ Pounding
☐ Dull aching   ☐ Burning   ☐ Sharp   ☐ Debilitating

Other:_____

ONSET

☐ Slow   ☐ Average   ☐ Rapid   ☐ Sudden

WHERE DOES IT HURT, EXACTLY?

OTHER SYMPTOMS

☐ Lightheaded   ☐ Dizziness   ☐ Confusion
☐ Light sensitivity   ☐ Sound sensitivity   ☐ Auras
☐ Muscle stiffness   ☐ Muscle burning   ☐ Muscle aches

HOW ARE YOU FEELING OVERALL?

Feeling sick?

Mood	① ② ③ ④ ⑤ ⑥ ⑦ ⑧ ⑨ ⑩	☐ Nope!
Energy levels	① ② ③ ④ ⑤ ⑥ ⑦ ⑧ ⑨ ⑩	☐ Yes...
Mental clarity	① ② ③ ④ ⑤ ⑥ ⑦ ⑧ ⑨ ⑩	

☐ Nausea   ☐ Diarrhea   ☐ Vomiting   ☐ Sore throat
☐ Congestion   ☐ Coughing   ☐ Chills   ☐ Fever

Other symptoms: _____

LAST NIGHT'S SLEEP

Hours of Sleep: _____   Sleep Quality: ① ② ③ ④ ⑤

WEATHER

☐ Hot   ☐ Mild   ☐ Cold   BM Pressure: _____

☐ Dry   ☐ Humid   ☐ Wet   Allergen Levels: _____

☐ Sunny   ☐ Cloudy

STRESS LEVELS

None	Low	Medium	High	Max	@$#%!

FOOD / DRINKS + NON-RELIEF MEDICATION / SUPPLEMENTS

item / meal	time	meds / supplements	dose	time

How many drinks?

water   → ① ② ③ ④ ⑤ ⑥ ⑦ ⑧ ⑨ ⑩

caffeine → ① ② ③ ④ ⑤ ⑥ ⑦ ⑧ ⑨ ⑩

alcohol → ① ② ③ ④ ⑤ ⑥ ⑦ ⑧ ⑨ ⑩

HORMONES

☐ Menstruating   ☐ Menopause   ☐ PMS   ☐ N/A | other

COMPUTER USE / READING

☐ None   ☐ Some   ☐ A lot   Total time: [   ]

☐ Sitting   ☐ Standing   ☐ Mixture   Breaks every: [   ]

PHYSICAL ACTIVITY

☐ None   ☐ Minimal   ☐ Some   ☐ Sweatin'   ☐ I'm beat

DETAILS: _____

RELIEF MEASURES

☐ Medication   ☐ Massage   ☐ Sleep   ☐ Exercise

☐ Water   ☐ Cold/Ice   ☐ Heat/Bath   ☐ Other

DETAILS: _____

DID IT WORK?   ☐ Nope   ☐ A bit   ☐ Mostly   ☐ 100%

Notes

Date:_____

START:	END:	DURATION:

| MIGRAINE | CLUSTER | SINUS | TMJ | TENSION |

PAIN LEVEL

1	2	3	4	5	6	7	8	9	10

Not too bad. *Well, I'm not enjoying this.* *Holy shit, make it stop!*

DETAILED DESCRIPTION

☐ Constant ☐ Squeezing ☐ Throbbing ☐ Pounding
☐ Dull aching ☐ Burning ☐ Sharp ☐ Debilitating

Other:_____

ONSET

☐ Slow ☐ Average ☐ Rapid ☐ Sudden

WHERE DOES IT HURT, EXACTLY?

OTHER SYMPTOMS

☐ Lightheaded ☐ Dizziness ☐ Confusion
☐ Light sensitivity ☐ Sound sensitivity ☐ Auras
☐ Muscle stiffness ☐ Muscle burning ☐ Muscle aches

HOW ARE YOU FEELING OVERALL?

Feeling sick?

Mood	① ② ③ ④ ⑤ ⑥ ⑦ ⑧ ⑨ ⑩
Energy levels	① ② ③ ④ ⑤ ⑥ ⑦ ⑧ ⑨ ⑩
Mental clarity	① ② ③ ④ ⑤ ⑥ ⑦ ⑧ ⑨ ⑩

☐ Nope!
☐ Yes...

☐ Nausea ☐ Diarrhea ☐ Vomiting ☐ Sore throat
☐ Congestion ☐ Coughing ☐ Chills ☐ Fever

Other symptoms:_____

LAST NIGHT'S SLEEP

Hours of Sleep: _____   Sleep Quality: ① ② ③ ④ ⑤

WEATHER

☐ Hot   ☐ Mild   ☐ Cold   BM Pressure: _____

☐ Dry   ☐ Humid   ☐ Wet   Allergen Levels: _____

☐ Sunny   ☐ Cloudy

STRESS LEVELS

None	Low	Medium	High	Max	@$#%!

FOOD / DRINKS + NON-RELIEF MEDICATION / SUPPLEMENTS

item / meal	time	meds / supplements	dose	time

How many drinks?

water   → ① ② ③ ④ ⑤ ⑥ ⑦ ⑧ ⑨ ⑩

caffeine → ① ② ③ ④ ⑤ ⑥ ⑦ ⑧ ⑨ ⑩

alcohol → ① ② ③ ④ ⑤ ⑥ ⑦ ⑧ ⑨ ⑩

HORMONES

☐ Menstruating   ☐ Menopause   ☐ PMS   ☐ N/A | other

COMPUTER USE / READING

☐ None   ☐ Some   ☐ A lot   Total time: [_____]

☐ Sitting   ☐ Standing   ☐ Mixture   Breaks every: [_____]

PHYSICAL ACTIVITY

☐ None   ☐ Minimal   ☐ Some   ☐ Sweatin'   ☐ I'm beat

DETAILS: _____

RELIEF MEASURES

☐ Medication   ☐ Massage   ☐ Sleep   ☐ Exercise

☐ Water   ☐ Cold/Ice   ☐ Heat/Bath   ☐ Other

DETAILS: _____

DID IT WORK?   ☐ Nope   ☐ A bit   ☐ Mostly   ☐ 100%

Notes

Date:_____

START:	END:	DURATION:

MIGRAINE

CLUSTER

SINUS

TMJ

TENSION

PAIN LEVEL

1	2	3	4	5	6	7	8	9	10

Not too bad.   *Well, I'm not enjoying this.*   *Holy shit, make it stop!*

DETAILED DESCRIPTION

☐ Constant   ☐ Squeezing   ☐ Throbbing   ☐ Pounding
☐ Dull aching   ☐ Burning   ☐ Sharp   ☐ Debilitating

Other:_____

ONSET

☐ Slow   ☐ Average   ☐ Rapid   ☐ Sudden

WHERE DOES IT HURT, EXACTLY?

OTHER SYMPTOMS

☐ Lightheaded   ☐ Dizziness   ☐ Confusion
☐ Light sensitivity   ☐ Sound sensitivity   ☐ Auras
☐ Muscle stiffness   ☐ Muscle burning   ☐ Muscle aches

HOW ARE YOU FEELING OVERALL?   Feeling sick?

Mood   ① ② ③ ④ ⑤ ⑥ ⑦ ⑧ ⑨ ⑩   ☐ Nope!

Energy levels ① ② ③ ④ ⑤ ⑥ ⑦ ⑧ ⑨ ⑩   ☐ Yes...

Mental clarity ① ② ③ ④ ⑤ ⑥ ⑦ ⑧ ⑨ ⑩

☐ Nausea   ☐ Diarrhea   ☐ Vomiting   ☐ Sore throat
☐ Congestion   ☐ Coughing   ☐ Chills   ☐ Fever

Other symptoms: _____

LAST NIGHT'S SLEEP

Hours of Sleep: _____   Sleep Quality: ① ② ③ ④ ⑤

WEATHER

☐ Hot   ☐ Mild   ☐ Cold   BM Pressure: _____

☐ Dry   ☐ Humid   ☐ Wet   Allergen Levels: _____

☐ Sunny   ☐ Cloudy

STRESS LEVELS

None	Low	Medium	High	Max	@$#%!

FOOD / DRINKS + NON-RELIEF MEDICATION / SUPPLEMENTS

item / meal	time	meds / supplements	dose	time

How many drinks?

water   ① ② ③ ④ ⑤ ⑥ ⑦ ⑧ ⑨ ⑩

caffeine ① ② ③ ④ ⑤ ⑥ ⑦ ⑧ ⑨ ⑩

alcohol ① ② ③ ④ ⑤ ⑥ ⑦ ⑧ ⑨ ⑩

HORMONES

☐ Menstruating ☐ Menopause ☐ PMS   ☐ N/A | other

COMPUTER USE / READING

☐ None   ☐ Some   ☐ A lot   Total time: [   ]

☐ Sitting   ☐ Standing   ☐ Mixture   Breaks every: [   ]

PHYSICAL ACTIVITY

☐ None   ☐ Minimal   ☐ Some   ☐ Sweatin'   ☐ I'm beat

DETAILS: _____

RELIEF MEASURES

☐ Medication   ☐ Massage   ☐ Sleep   ☐ Exercise

☐ Water   ☐ Cold/Ice   ☐ Heat/Bath ☐ Other

DETAILS: _____

DID IT WORK?   ☐ Nope   ☐ A bit   ☐ Mostly   ☐ 100%

Notes

Date:_____

START:	END:	DURATION:

| MIGRAINE | CLUSTER | SINUS | TMJ | TENSION |

PAIN LEVEL

1	2	3	4	5	6	7	8	9	10

Not too bad.　　　*Well, I'm not enjoying this.*　　　*Holy shit, make it stop!*

DETAILED DESCRIPTION

☐ Constant　☐ Squeezing　☐ Throbbing　☐ Pounding
☐ Dull aching　☐ Burning　☐ Sharp　☐ Debilitating

Other:_____

ONSET

☐ Slow　　☐ Average　　☐ Rapid　　☐ Sudden

WHERE DOES IT HURT, EXACTLY?

OTHER SYMPTOMS

☐ Lightheaded　　☐ Dizziness　　☐ Confusion
☐ Light sensitivity　☐ Sound sensitivity　☐ Auras
☐ Muscle stiffness　☐ Muscle burning　☐ Muscle aches

HOW ARE YOU FEELING OVERALL?　　　Feeling sick?

Mood	① ② ③ ④ ⑤ ⑥ ⑦ ⑧ ⑨ ⑩	☐ Nope!
Energy levels	① ② ③ ④ ⑤ ⑥ ⑦ ⑧ ⑨ ⑩	☐ Yes...
Mental clarity	① ② ③ ④ ⑤ ⑥ ⑦ ⑧ ⑨ ⑩	

☐ Nausea　　☐ Diarrhea　　☐ Vomiting　　☐ Sore throat
☐ Congestion　☐ Coughing　☐ Chills　　☐ Fever

Other symptoms: _____

LAST NIGHT'S SLEEP

Hours of Sleep: _____   Sleep Quality: ① ② ③ ④ ⑤

WEATHER

☐ Hot   ☐ Mild   ☐ Cold   BM Pressure: _____

☐ Dry   ☐ Humid   ☐ Wet   Allergen Levels: _____

☐ Sunny   ☐ Cloudy

STRESS LEVELS

None	Low	Medium	High	Max	@$#%!

FOOD / DRINKS + NON-RELIEF MEDICATION / SUPPLEMENTS

item / meal	time	meds / supplements	dose	time

How many drinks?

water → ① ② ③ ④ ⑤ ⑥ ⑦ ⑧ ⑨ ⑩

caffeine → ① ② ③ ④ ⑤ ⑥ ⑦ ⑧ ⑨ ⑩

alcohol → ① ② ③ ④ ⑤ ⑥ ⑦ ⑧ ⑨ ⑩

HORMONES

☐ Menstruating   ☐ Menopause   ☐ PMS   ☐ N/A | other

COMPUTER USE / READING

☐ None   ☐ Some   ☐ A lot   Total time: _____

☐ Sitting   ☐ Standing   ☐ Mixture   Breaks every: _____

PHYSICAL ACTIVITY

☐ None   ☐ Minimal   ☐ Some   ☐ Sweatin'   ☐ I'm beat

DETAILS: _____

RELIEF MEASURES

☐ Medication   ☐ Massage   ☐ Sleep   ☐ Exercise

☐ Water   ☐ Cold/Ice   ☐ Heat/Bath   ☐ Other

DETAILS: _____

DID IT WORK?   ☐ Nope   ☐ A bit   ☐ Mostly   ☐ 100%

Notes

Date:_____

START:	END:	DURATION:

MIGRAINE	CLUSTER	SINUS	TMJ	TENSION

PAIN LEVEL

1	2	3	4	5	6	7	8	9	10

Not too bad.   *Well, I'm not enjoying this.*   *Holy shit, make it stop!*

DETAILED DESCRIPTION

☐ Constant ☐ Squeezing ☐ Throbbing ☐ Pounding
☐ Dull aching ☐ Burning ☐ Sharp ☐ Debilitating

Other:_____

ONSET

☐ Slow ☐ Average ☐ Rapid ☐ Sudden

WHERE DOES IT HURT, EXACTLY?

OTHER SYMPTOMS

☐ Lightheaded ☐ Dizziness ☐ Confusion
☐ Light sensitivity ☐ Sound sensitivity ☐ Auras
☐ Muscle stiffness ☐ Muscle burning ☐ Muscle aches

HOW ARE YOU FEELING OVERALL?

Feeling sick?

Mood ① ② ③ ④ ⑤ ⑥ ⑦ ⑧ ⑨ ⑩   ☐ Nope!

Energy levels ① ② ③ ④ ⑤ ⑥ ⑦ ⑧ ⑨ ⑩   ☐ Yes...

Mental clarity ① ② ③ ④ ⑤ ⑥ ⑦ ⑧ ⑨ ⑩

☐ Nausea ☐ Diarrhea ☐ Vomiting ☐ Sore throat
☐ Congestion ☐ Coughing ☐ Chills ☐ Fever

Other symptoms: _____

LAST NIGHT'S SLEEP

Hours of Sleep: _____   Sleep Quality: ① ② ③ ④ ⑤

WEATHER

☐ Hot   ☐ Mild   ☐ Cold   BM Pressure: _____

☐ Dry   ☐ Humid   ☐ Wet   Allergen Levels: _____

☐ Sunny   ☐ Cloudy

STRESS LEVELS

None	Low	Medium	High	Max	@$#%!

FOOD / DRINKS + NON-RELIEF MEDICATION / SUPPLEMENTS

item / meal	time	meds / supplements	dose	time

How many drinks?

water ⟹ ① ② ③ ④ ⑤ ⑥ ⑦ ⑧ ⑨ ⑩

caffeine ⟹ ① ② ③ ④ ⑤ ⑥ ⑦ ⑧ ⑨ ⑩

alcohol ⟹ ① ② ③ ④ ⑤ ⑥ ⑦ ⑧ ⑨ ⑩

HORMONES

☐ Menstruating   ☐ Menopause   ☐ PMS   ☐ N/A | other

COMPUTER USE / READING

☐ None   ☐ Some   ☐ A lot   Total time: [   ]

☐ Sitting   ☐ Standing   ☐ Mixture   Breaks every: [   ]

PHYSICAL ACTIVITY

☐ None   ☐ Minimal   ☐ Some   ☐ Sweatin'   ☐ I'm beat

DETAILS: _____

RELIEF MEASURES

☐ Medication   ☐ Massage   ☐ Sleep   ☐ Exercise

☐ Water   ☐ Cold/Ice   ☐ Heat/Bath   ☐ Other

DETAILS: _____

DID IT WORK?   ☐ Nope   ☐ A bit   ☐ Mostly   ☐ 100%

Notes

Date:_____

START:	END:	DURATION:

MIGRAINE	CLUSTER	SINUS	TMJ	TENSION

PAIN LEVEL

1	2	3	4	5	6	7	8	9	10

Not too bad.　　　*Well, I'm not enjoying this.*　　　*Holy shit, make it stop!*

DETAILED DESCRIPTION

☐ Constant　　☐ Squeezing　　☐ Throbbing　　☐ Pounding
☐ Dull aching　☐ Burning　　　☐ Sharp　　　☐ Debilitating

Other:_____

ONSET

☐ Slow　　　☐ Average　　☐ Rapid　　☐ Sudden

WHERE DOES IT HURT, EXACTLY?

OTHER SYMPTOMS

☐ Lightheaded　　　☐ Dizziness　　　☐ Confusion
☐ Light sensitivity　☐ Sound sensitivity　☐ Auras
☐ Muscle stiffness　☐ Muscle burning　☐ Muscle aches

HOW ARE YOU FEELING OVERALL?　　　　Feeling sick?

Mood	① ② ③ ④ ⑤ ⑥ ⑦ ⑧ ⑨ ⑩	☐ Nope!
Energy levels	① ② ③ ④ ⑤ ⑥ ⑦ ⑧ ⑨ ⑩	☐ Yes...
Mental clarity	① ② ③ ④ ⑤ ⑥ ⑦ ⑧ ⑨ ⑩	

☐ Nausea　　☐ Diarrhea　　☐ Vomiting　　☐ Sore throat
☐ Congestion　☐ Coughing　　☐ Chills　　　☐ Fever

Other symptoms: _____

LAST NIGHT'S SLEEP

Hours of Sleep: _____ Sleep Quality: ① ② ③ ④ ⑤

WEATHER

☐ Hot   ☐ Mild   ☐ Cold   BM Pressure: _____

☐ Dry   ☐ Humid   ☐ Wet   Allergen Levels: _____

☐ Sunny   ☐ Cloudy

STRESS LEVELS

None	Low	Medium	High	Max	@$#%!

FOOD / DRINKS + NON-RELIEF MEDICATION / SUPPLEMENTS

item / meal	time	meds / supplements	dose	time

How many drinks?

water   ⟹ ① ② ③ ④ ⑤ ⑥ ⑦ ⑧ ⑨ ⑩

caffeine ⟹ ① ② ③ ④ ⑤ ⑥ ⑦ ⑧ ⑨ ⑩

alcohol ⟹ ① ② ③ ④ ⑤ ⑥ ⑦ ⑧ ⑨ ⑩

HORMONES

☐ Menstruating   ☐ Menopause   ☐ PMS   ☐ N/A | other

COMPUTER USE / READING

☐ None   ☐ Some   ☐ A lot   Total time: [   ]

☐ Sitting   ☐ Standing   ☐ Mixture   Breaks every: [   ]

PHYSICAL ACTIVITY

☐ None   ☐ Minimal   ☐ Some   ☐ Sweatin'   ☐ I'm beat

DETAILS: _____

RELIEF MEASURES

☐ Medication   ☐ Massage   ☐ Sleep   ☐ Exercise

☐ Water   ☐ Cold/Ice   ☐ Heat/Bath   ☐ Other

DETAILS: _____

DID IT WORK?   ☐ Nope   ☐ A bit   ☐ Mostly   ☐ 100%

Notes

Date:_____

START:	END:	DURATION:

MIGRAINE	CLUSTER	SINUS	TMJ	TENSION

PAIN LEVEL

1	2	3	4	5	6	7	8	9	10

Not too bad.   *Well, I'm not enjoying this.*   *Holy shit, make it stop!*

DETAILED DESCRIPTION

☐ Constant ☐ Squeezing ☐ Throbbing ☐ Pounding
☐ Dull aching ☐ Burning ☐ Sharp ☐ Debilitating

Other:_____

ONSET

☐ Slow ☐ Average ☐ Rapid ☐ Sudden

WHERE DOES IT HURT, EXACTLY?

OTHER SYMPTOMS

☐ Lightheaded ☐ Dizziness ☐ Confusion
☐ Light sensitivity ☐ Sound sensitivity ☐ Auras
☐ Muscle stiffness ☐ Muscle burning ☐ Muscle aches

HOW ARE YOU FEELING OVERALL?

Feeling sick?

Mood	① ② ③ ④ ⑤ ⑥ ⑦ ⑧ ⑨ ⑩	☐ Nope!
Energy levels	① ② ③ ④ ⑤ ⑥ ⑦ ⑧ ⑨ ⑩	☐ Yes...
Mental clarity	① ② ③ ④ ⑤ ⑥ ⑦ ⑧ ⑨ ⑩	

☐ Nausea ☐ Diarrhea ☐ Vomiting ☐ Sore throat
☐ Congestion ☐ Coughing ☐ Chills ☐ Fever

Other symptoms: _____

LAST NIGHT'S SLEEP

Hours of Sleep: _____   Sleep Quality: ① ② ③ ④ ⑤

WEATHER

☐ Hot   ☐ Mild   ☐ Cold   BM Pressure: _____

☐ Dry   ☐ Humid   ☐ Wet   Allergen Levels: _____

☐ Sunny   ☐ Cloudy

STRESS LEVELS

None	Low	Medium	High	Max	@$#%!

FOOD / DRINKS + NON-RELIEF MEDICATION / SUPPLEMENTS

item / meal	time	meds / supplements	dose	time

How many drinks?

water   ① ② ③ ④ ⑤ ⑥ ⑦ ⑧ ⑨ ⑩

caffeine ① ② ③ ④ ⑤ ⑥ ⑦ ⑧ ⑨ ⑩

alcohol   ① ② ③ ④ ⑤ ⑥ ⑦ ⑧ ⑨ ⑩

HORMONES

☐ Menstruating   ☐ Menopause   ☐ PMS   ☐ N/A | other

COMPUTER USE / READING

☐ None   ☐ Some   ☐ A lot   Total time: [   ]

☐ Sitting   ☐ Standing   ☐ Mixture   Breaks every: [   ]

PHYSICAL ACTIVITY

☐ None   ☐ Minimal   ☐ Some   ☐ Sweatin'   ☐ I'm beat

DETAILS: _____

RELIEF MEASURES

☐ Medication   ☐ Massage   ☐ Sleep   ☐ Exercise

☐ Water   ☐ Cold/Ice   ☐ Heat/Bath   ☐ Other

DETAILS: _____

DID IT WORK?   ☐ Nope   ☐ A bit   ☐ Mostly   ☐ 100%

Notes

Date:_____

START:	END:	DURATION:

| MIGRAINE | CLUSTER | SINUS | TMJ | TENSION |

PAIN LEVEL

1	2	3	4	5	6	7	8	9	10

Not too bad.   *Well, I'm not enjoying this.*   *Holy shit, make it stop!*

DETAILED DESCRIPTION

☐ Constant   ☐ Squeezing   ☐ Throbbing   ☐ Pounding
☐ Dull aching   ☐ Burning   ☐ Sharp   ☐ Debilitating

Other:_____

ONSET

☐ Slow   ☐ Average   ☐ Rapid   ☐ Sudden

WHERE DOES IT HURT, EXACTLY?

OTHER SYMPTOMS

☐ Lightheaded   ☐ Dizziness   ☐ Confusion
☐ Light sensitivity   ☐ Sound sensitivity   ☐ Auras
☐ Muscle stiffness   ☐ Muscle burning   ☐ Muscle aches

HOW ARE YOU FEELING OVERALL?

Feeling sick?

Mood   ① ② ③ ④ ⑤ ⑥ ⑦ ⑧ ⑨ ⑩   ☐ Nope!
Energy levels   ① ② ③ ④ ⑤ ⑥ ⑦ ⑧ ⑨ ⑩   ☐ Yes...
Mental clarity   ① ② ③ ④ ⑤ ⑥ ⑦ ⑧ ⑨ ⑩

☐ Nausea   ☐ Diarrhea   ☐ Vomiting   ☐ Sore throat
☐ Congestion   ☐ Coughing   ☐ Chills   ☐ Fever

Other symptoms: _____

LAST NIGHT'S SLEEP

Hours of Sleep: _____   Sleep Quality: ① ② ③ ④ ⑤

WEATHER

☐ Hot   ☐ Mild   ☐ Cold   BM Pressure: _____

☐ Dry   ☐ Humid   ☐ Wet   Allergen Levels: _____

☐ Sunny   ☐ Cloudy

STRESS LEVELS

None	Low	Medium	High	Max	@$#%!

FOOD / DRINKS + NON-RELIEF MEDICATION / SUPPLEMENTS

item / meal	time	meds / supplements	dose	time

How many drinks?

water → ① ② ③ ④ ⑤ ⑥ ⑦ ⑧ ⑨ ⑩

caffeine → ① ② ③ ④ ⑤ ⑥ ⑦ ⑧ ⑨ ⑩

alcohol → ① ② ③ ④ ⑤ ⑥ ⑦ ⑧ ⑨ ⑩

HORMONES

☐ Menstruating   ☐ Menopause   ☐ PMS   ☐ N/A | other

COMPUTER USE / READING

☐ None   ☐ Some   ☐ A lot   Total time: [____]

☐ Sitting   ☐ Standing ☐ Mixture   Breaks every: [____]

PHYSICAL ACTIVITY

☐ None   ☐ Minimal   ☐ Some   ☐ Sweatin'   ☐ I'm beat

DETAILS: _____

RELIEF MEASURES

☐ Medication   ☐ Massage   ☐ Sleep   ☐ Exercise

☐ Water   ☐ Cold/Ice   ☐ Heat/Bath ☐ Other

DETAILS: _____

DID IT WORK?   ☐ Nope   ☐ A bit   ☐ Mostly   ☐ 100%

Notes

Date: _____

START:	END:	DURATION:

MIGRAINE CLUSTER SINUS TMJ TENSION

PAIN LEVEL

1	2	3	4	5	6	7	8	9	10

Not too bad. *Well, I'm not enjoying this.* *Holy shit, make it stop!*

DETAILED DESCRIPTION

☐ Constant ☐ Squeezing ☐ Throbbing ☐ Pounding
☐ Dull aching ☐ Burning ☐ Sharp ☐ Debilitating

Other:_____

ONSET

☐ Slow ☐ Average ☐ Rapid ☐ Sudden

WHERE DOES IT HURT, EXACTLY?

OTHER SYMPTOMS

☐ Lightheaded ☐ Dizziness ☐ Confusion
☐ Light sensitivity ☐ Sound sensitivity ☐ Auras
☐ Muscle stiffness ☐ Muscle burning ☐ Muscle aches

HOW ARE YOU FEELING OVERALL?

Feeling sick?

Mood ① ② ③ ④ ⑤ ⑥ ⑦ ⑧ ⑨ ⑩ ☐ Nope!

Energy levels ① ② ③ ④ ⑤ ⑥ ⑦ ⑧ ⑨ ⑩ ☐ Yes...

Mental clarity ① ② ③ ④ ⑤ ⑥ ⑦ ⑧ ⑨ ⑩

☐ Nausea ☐ Diarrhea ☐ Vomiting ☐ Sore throat
☐ Congestion ☐ Coughing ☐ Chills ☐ Fever

Other symptoms: _____

LAST NIGHT'S SLEEP

Hours of Sleep: _____   Sleep Quality: ① ② ③ ④ ⑤

WEATHER

☐ Hot   ☐ Mild   ☐ Cold   BM Pressure: _____

☐ Dry   ☐ Humid   ☐ Wet   Allergen Levels: _____

☐ Sunny   ☐ Cloudy

STRESS LEVELS

None	Low	Medium	High	Max	@$#%!

FOOD / DRINKS + NON-RELIEF MEDICATION / SUPPLEMENTS

item / meal	time	meds / supplements	dose	time

How many drinks?

water   ➜ ① ② ③ ④ ⑤ ⑥ ⑦ ⑧ ⑨ ⑩
caffeine ➜ ① ② ③ ④ ⑤ ⑥ ⑦ ⑧ ⑨ ⑩
alcohol ➜ ① ② ③ ④ ⑤ ⑥ ⑦ ⑧ ⑨ ⑩

HORMONES

☐ Menstruating ☐ Menopause ☐ PMS   ☐ N/A | other

COMPUTER USE / READING

☐ None   ☐ Some   ☐ A lot   Total time: [____]

☐ Sitting   ☐ Standing   ☐ Mixture   Breaks every: [____]

PHYSICAL ACTIVITY

☐ None   ☐ Minimal   ☐ Some   ☐ Sweatin'   ☐ I'm beat

DETAILS: _____

RELIEF MEASURES

☐ Medication ☐ Massage   ☐ Sleep   ☐ Exercise

☐ Water   ☐ Cold/Ice   ☐ Heat/Bath   ☐ Other

DETAILS: _____

DID IT WORK?   ☐ Nope   ☐ A bit   ☐ Mostly   ☐ 100%

Notes

Date:_____

START:	END:	DURATION:

MIGRAINE　　CLUSTER　　SINUS　　TMJ　　TENSION

PAIN LEVEL

1	2	3	4	5	6	7	8	9	10

Not too bad.　　*Well, I'm not enjoying this.*　　*Holy shit, make it stop!*

DETAILED DESCRIPTION

☐ Constant　　☐ Squeezing　　☐ Throbbing　　☐ Pounding
☐ Dull aching　☐ Burning　　☐ Sharp　　☐ Debilitating

Other:_____

ONSET

☐ Slow　　☐ Average　　☐ Rapid　　☐ Sudden

WHERE DOES IT HURT, EXACTLY?

OTHER SYMPTOMS

☐ Lightheaded　　☐ Dizziness　　☐ Confusion
☐ Light sensitivity　☐ Sound sensitivity　☐ Auras
☐ Muscle stiffness　☐ Muscle burning　☐ Muscle aches

HOW ARE YOU FEELING OVERALL?

Feeling sick?

Mood	① ② ③ ④ ⑤ ⑥ ⑦ ⑧ ⑨ ⑩	☐ Nope!
Energy levels	① ② ③ ④ ⑤ ⑥ ⑦ ⑧ ⑨ ⑩	☐ Yes...
Mental clarity	① ② ③ ④ ⑤ ⑥ ⑦ ⑧ ⑨ ⑩	

☐ Nausea　　☐ Diarrhea　　☐ Vomiting　　☐ Sore throat
☐ Congestion　☐ Coughing　　☐ Chills　　☐ Fever

Other symptoms:_____

LAST NIGHT'S SLEEP

Hours of Sleep: _____   Sleep Quality: ① ② ③ ④ ⑤

WEATHER

☐ Hot   ☐ Mild   ☐ Cold   BM Pressure: _____

☐ Dry   ☐ Humid   ☐ Wet   Allergen Levels: _____

☐ Sunny   ☐ Cloudy

STRESS LEVELS

None	Low	Medium	High	Max	@$#%!

FOOD / DRINKS + NON-RELIEF MEDICATION / SUPPLEMENTS

item / meal	time	meds / supplements	dose	time

How many drinks?

water	⟶	① ② ③ ④ ⑤ ⑥ ⑦ ⑧ ⑨ ⑩
caffeine	⟶	① ② ③ ④ ⑤ ⑥ ⑦ ⑧ ⑨ ⑩
alcohol	⟶	① ② ③ ④ ⑤ ⑥ ⑦ ⑧ ⑨ ⑩

HORMONES

☐ Menstruating   ☐ Menopause   ☐ PMS   ☐ N/A | other

COMPUTER USE / READING

☐ None   ☐ Some   ☐ A lot   Total time: [   ]

☐ Sitting   ☐ Standing   ☐ Mixture   Breaks every: [   ]

PHYSICAL ACTIVITY

☐ None   ☐ Minimal   ☐ Some   ☐ Sweatin'   ☐ I'm beat

DETAILS: _____

RELIEF MEASURES

☐ Medication   ☐ Massage   ☐ Sleep   ☐ Exercise

☐ Water   ☐ Cold/Ice   ☐ Heat/Bath   ☐ Other

DETAILS: _____

DID IT WORK?   ☐ Nope   ☐ A bit   ☐ Mostly   ☐ 100%

Notes

Date: _ _ _ _ _ _ _ _

START:	END:	DURATION:

MIGRAINE

CLUSTER

SINUS

TMJ

TENSION

PAIN LEVEL

1	2	3	4	5	6	7	8	9	10

Not too bad. *Well, I'm not enjoying this.* *Holy shit, make it stop!*

DETAILED DESCRIPTION

☐ Constant ☐ Squeezing ☐ Throbbing ☐ Pounding
☐ Dull aching ☐ Burning ☐ Sharp ☐ Debilitating

Other:_____

ONSET

☐ Slow ☐ Average ☐ Rapid ☐ Sudden

WHERE DOES IT HURT, EXACTLY?

OTHER SYMPTOMS

☐ Lightheaded ☐ Dizziness ☐ Confusion
☐ Light sensitivity ☐ Sound sensitivity ☐ Auras
☐ Muscle stiffness ☐ Muscle burning ☐ Muscle aches

HOW ARE YOU FEELING OVERALL?

Feeling sick?

Mood ① ② ③ ④ ⑤ ⑥ ⑦ ⑧ ⑨ ⑩ ☐ Nope!

Energy levels ① ② ③ ④ ⑤ ⑥ ⑦ ⑧ ⑨ ⑩ ☐ Yes...

Mental clarity ① ② ③ ④ ⑤ ⑥ ⑦ ⑧ ⑨ ⑩

☐ Nausea ☐ Diarrhea ☐ Vomiting ☐ Sore throat
☐ Congestion ☐ Coughing ☐ Chills ☐ Fever

Other symptoms: _____

LAST NIGHT'S SLEEP

Hours of Sleep: _____   Sleep Quality: ① ② ③ ④ ⑤

WEATHER

☐ Hot   ☐ Mild   ☐ Cold   BM Pressure: _____

☐ Dry   ☐ Humid   ☐ Wet   Allergen Levels: _____

☐ Sunny   ☐ Cloudy

STRESS LEVELS

None	Low	Medium	High	Max	@$#%!

FOOD / DRINKS + NON-RELIEF MEDICATION / SUPPLEMENTS

item / meal	time	meds / supplements	dose	time

How many drinks?

water → ① ② ③ ④ ⑤ ⑥ ⑦ ⑧ ⑨ ⑩

caffeine → ① ② ③ ④ ⑤ ⑥ ⑦ ⑧ ⑨ ⑩

alcohol → ① ② ③ ④ ⑤ ⑥ ⑦ ⑧ ⑨ ⑩

HORMONES

☐ Menstruating   ☐ Menopause   ☐ PMS   ☐ N/A | other

COMPUTER USE / READING

☐ None   ☐ Some   ☐ A lot   Total time: [   ]

☐ Sitting   ☐ Standing   ☐ Mixture   Breaks every: [   ]

PHYSICAL ACTIVITY

☐ None   ☐ Minimal   ☐ Some   ☐ Sweatin'   ☐ I'm beat

DETAILS: _____

RELIEF MEASURES

☐ Medication   ☐ Massage   ☐ Sleep   ☐ Exercise

☐ Water   ☐ Cold/Ice   ☐ Heat/Bath   ☐ Other

DETAILS: _____

DID IT WORK?   ☐ Nope   ☐ A bit   ☐ Mostly   ☐ 100%

Notes

Date:_____

START:	END:	DURATION:

| MIGRAINE | CLUSTER | SINUS | TMJ | TENSION |

PAIN LEVEL

1	2	3	4	5	6	7	8	9	10

Not too bad. *Well, I'm not enjoying this.* *Holy shit, make it stop!*

DETAILED DESCRIPTION

☐ Constant ☐ Squeezing ☐ Throbbing ☐ Pounding
☐ Dull aching ☐ Burning ☐ Sharp ☐ Debilitating

Other:_____

ONSET

☐ Slow ☐ Average ☐ Rapid ☐ Sudden

WHERE DOES IT HURT, EXACTLY?

OTHER SYMPTOMS

☐ Lightheaded ☐ Dizziness ☐ Confusion
☐ Light sensitivity ☐ Sound sensitivity ☐ Auras
☐ Muscle stiffness ☐ Muscle burning ☐ Muscle aches

HOW ARE YOU FEELING OVERALL?   Feeling sick?

Mood	① ② ③ ④ ⑤ ⑥ ⑦ ⑧ ⑨ ⑩	☐ Nope!
Energy levels	① ② ③ ④ ⑤ ⑥ ⑦ ⑧ ⑨ ⑩	☐ Yes...
Mental clarity	① ② ③ ④ ⑤ ⑥ ⑦ ⑧ ⑨ ⑩	

☐ Nausea ☐ Diarrhea ☐ Vomiting ☐ Sore throat
☐ Congestion ☐ Coughing ☐ Chills ☐ Fever

Other symptoms: _____

LAST NIGHT'S SLEEP

Hours of Sleep: _____   Sleep Quality: ① ② ③ ④ ⑤

WEATHER

☐ Hot   ☐ Mild   ☐ Cold   BM Pressure: _____

☐ Dry   ☐ Humid   ☐ Wet   Allergen Levels: _____

☐ Sunny   ☐ Cloudy

STRESS LEVELS

None	Low	Medium	High	Max	@$#%!

FOOD / DRINKS + NON-RELIEF MEDICATION / SUPPLEMENTS

item / meal	time	meds / supplements	dose	time

How many drinks?

water → ① ② ③ ④ ⑤ ⑥ ⑦ ⑧ ⑨ ⑩

caffeine → ① ② ③ ④ ⑤ ⑥ ⑦ ⑧ ⑨ ⑩

alcohol → ① ② ③ ④ ⑤ ⑥ ⑦ ⑧ ⑨ ⑩

HORMONES

☐ Menstruating   ☐ Menopause   ☐ PMS   ☐ N/A | other

COMPUTER USE / READING

☐ None   ☐ Some   ☐ A lot   Total time: [____]

☐ Sitting   ☐ Standing ☐ Mixture   Breaks every: [____]

PHYSICAL ACTIVITY

☐ None   ☐ Minimal   ☐ Some   ☐ Sweatin'   ☐ I'm beat

DETAILS: _____

RELIEF MEASURES

☐ Medication   ☐ Massage   ☐ Sleep   ☐ Exercise

☐ Water   ☐ Cold/Ice   ☐ Heat/Bath   ☐ Other

DETAILS: _____

DID IT WORK?   ☐ Nope   ☐ A bit   ☐ Mostly   ☐ 100%

Notes

Date:_____

START:	END:	DURATION:

MIGRAINE	CLUSTER	SINUS	TMJ	TENSION

PAIN LEVEL

1	2	3	4	5	6	7	8	9	10

Not too bad.   *Well, I'm not enjoying this.*   *Holy shit, make it stop!*

DETAILED DESCRIPTION

☐ Constant   ☐ Squeezing   ☐ Throbbing   ☐ Pounding
☐ Dull aching   ☐ Burning   ☐ Sharp   ☐ Debilitating

Other:_____

ONSET

☐ Slow   ☐ Average   ☐ Rapid   ☐ Sudden

WHERE DOES IT HURT, EXACTLY?

OTHER SYMPTOMS

☐ Lightheaded   ☐ Dizziness   ☐ Confusion
☐ Light sensitivity   ☐ Sound sensitivity   ☐ Auras
☐ Muscle stiffness   ☐ Muscle burning   ☐ Muscle aches

HOW ARE YOU FEELING OVERALL?   Feeling sick?

Mood	① ② ③ ④ ⑤ ⑥ ⑦ ⑧ ⑨ ⑩	☐ Nope!
Energy levels	① ② ③ ④ ⑤ ⑥ ⑦ ⑧ ⑨ ⑩	☐ Yes...
Mental clarity	① ② ③ ④ ⑤ ⑥ ⑦ ⑧ ⑨ ⑩	

☐ Nausea   ☐ Diarrhea   ☐ Vomiting   ☐ Sore throat
☐ Congestion   ☐ Coughing   ☐ Chills   ☐ Fever

Other symptoms: _____

LAST NIGHT'S SLEEP

Hours of Sleep: _____   Sleep Quality: ① ② ③ ④ ⑤

WEATHER

☐ Hot   ☐ Mild   ☐ Cold   BM Pressure: _____

☐ Dry   ☐ Humid   ☐ Wet   Allergen Levels: _____

☐ Sunny   ☐ Cloudy

STRESS LEVELS

None	Low	Medium	High	Max	@$#%!

FOOD / DRINKS + NON-RELIEF MEDICATION / SUPPLEMENTS

item / meal	time	meds / supplements	dose	time

How many drinks?

water   ① ② ③ ④ ⑤ ⑥ ⑦ ⑧ ⑨ ⑩

caffeine ① ② ③ ④ ⑤ ⑥ ⑦ ⑧ ⑨ ⑩

alcohol ① ② ③ ④ ⑤ ⑥ ⑦ ⑧ ⑨ ⑩

HORMONES

☐ Menstruating   ☐ Menopause   ☐ PMS   ☐ N/A | other

COMPUTER USE / READING

☐ None   ☐ Some   ☐ A lot   Total time: _____

☐ Sitting   ☐ Standing   ☐ Mixture   Breaks every: _____

PHYSICAL ACTIVITY

☐ None   ☐ Minimal   ☐ Some   ☐ Sweatin'   ☐ I'm beat

DETAILS: _____

RELIEF MEASURES

☐ Medication   ☐ Massage   ☐ Sleep   ☐ Exercise

☐ Water   ☐ Cold/Ice   ☐ Heat/Bath   ☐ Other

DETAILS: _____

DID IT WORK?   ☐ Nope   ☐ A bit   ☐ Mostly   ☐ 100%

Notes

Date:_____

START:	END:	DURATION:

| MIGRAINE | CLUSTER | SINUS | TMJ | TENSION |

PAIN LEVEL

1	2	3	4	5	6	7	8	9	10

Not too bad.   *Well, I'm not enjoying this.*   *Holy shit, make it stop!*

DETAILED DESCRIPTION

☐ Constant   ☐ Squeezing   ☐ Throbbing   ☐ Pounding
☐ Dull aching ☐ Burning   ☐ Sharp   ☐ Debilitating

Other:_____

ONSET

☐ Slow   ☐ Average   ☐ Rapid   ☐ Sudden

WHERE DOES IT HURT, EXACTLY?

OTHER SYMPTOMS

☐ Lightheaded   ☐ Dizziness   ☐ Confusion
☐ Light sensitivity ☐ Sound sensitivity ☐ Auras
☐ Muscle stiffness ☐ Muscle burning   ☐ Muscle aches

HOW ARE YOU FEELING OVERALL?

Feeling sick?

Mood ① ② ③ ④ ⑤ ⑥ ⑦ ⑧ ⑨ ⑩   ☐ Nope!

Energy levels ① ② ③ ④ ⑤ ⑥ ⑦ ⑧ ⑨ ⑩   ☐ Yes...

Mental clarity ① ② ③ ④ ⑤ ⑥ ⑦ ⑧ ⑨ ⑩

☐ Nausea   ☐ Diarrhea   ☐ Vomiting   ☐ Sore throat
☐ Congestion   ☐ Coughing   ☐ Chills   ☐ Fever

Other symptoms: _____

LAST NIGHT'S SLEEP

Hours of Sleep: _____   Sleep Quality: ① ② ③ ④ ⑤

WEATHER

☐ Hot   ☐ Mild   ☐ Cold   BM Pressure: _____
☐ Dry   ☐ Humid   ☐ Wet   Allergen Levels: _____
☐ Sunny   ☐ Cloudy

STRESS LEVELS

None	Low	Medium	High	Max	@$#%!

FOOD / DRINKS + NON-RELIEF MEDICATION / SUPPLEMENTS

item / meal	time	meds / supplements	dose	time

How many drinks?

water ⟹ ① ② ③ ④ ⑤ ⑥ ⑦ ⑧ ⑨ ⑩
caffeine ⟹ ① ② ③ ④ ⑤ ⑥ ⑦ ⑧ ⑨ ⑩
alcohol ⟹ ① ② ③ ④ ⑤ ⑥ ⑦ ⑧ ⑨ ⑩

HORMONES

☐ Menstruating   ☐ Menopause   ☐ PMS   ☐ N/A | other

COMPUTER USE / READING

☐ None   ☐ Some   ☐ A lot   Total time: [   ]
☐ Sitting   ☐ Standing   ☐ Mixture   Breaks every: [   ]

PHYSICAL ACTIVITY

☐ None   ☐ Minimal   ☐ Some   ☐ Sweatin'   ☐ I'm beat
DETAILS: _____

RELIEF MEASURES

☐ Medication   ☐ Massage   ☐ Sleep   ☐ Exercise
☐ Water   ☐ Cold/Ice   ☐ Heat/Bath   ☐ Other
DETAILS: _____

DID IT WORK?   ☐ Nope   ☐ A bit   ☐ Mostly   ☐ 100%

Notes

Date:_____

START:	END:	DURATION:

| MIGRAINE | CLUSTER | SINUS | TMJ | TENSION |

PAIN LEVEL

1	2	3	4	5	6	7	8	9	10

Not too bad.   *Well, I'm not enjoying this.*   *Holy shit, make it stop!*

DETAILED DESCRIPTION

☐ Constant   ☐ Squeezing   ☐ Throbbing   ☐ Pounding
☐ Dull aching   ☐ Burning   ☐ Sharp   ☐ Debilitating

Other:_____

ONSET

☐ Slow   ☐ Average   ☐ Rapid   ☐ Sudden

WHERE DOES IT HURT, EXACTLY?

OTHER SYMPTOMS

☐ Lightheaded   ☐ Dizziness   ☐ Confusion
☐ Light sensitivity   ☐ Sound sensitivity   ☐ Auras
☐ Muscle stiffness   ☐ Muscle burning   ☐ Muscle aches

HOW ARE YOU FEELING OVERALL?   Feeling sick?

Mood	① ② ③ ④ ⑤ ⑥ ⑦ ⑧ ⑨ ⑩	☐ Nope!
Energy levels	① ② ③ ④ ⑤ ⑥ ⑦ ⑧ ⑨ ⑩	☐ Yes...
Mental clarity	① ② ③ ④ ⑤ ⑥ ⑦ ⑧ ⑨ ⑩	

☐ Nausea   ☐ Diarrhea   ☐ Vomiting   ☐ Sore throat
☐ Congestion   ☐ Coughing   ☐ Chills   ☐ Fever

Other symptoms: _____

LAST NIGHT'S SLEEP

Hours of Sleep: _____ Sleep Quality: ① ② ③ ④ ⑤

WEATHER

☐ Hot   ☐ Mild   ☐ Cold   BM Pressure: _____

☐ Dry   ☐ Humid   ☐ Wet   Allergen Levels: _____

☐ Sunny   ☐ Cloudy

STRESS LEVELS

| None | Low | Medium | High | Max | @$#%! |

FOOD / DRINKS + NON-RELIEF MEDICATION / SUPPLEMENTS

item / meal	time	meds / supplements	dose	time

How many drinks?

water ⟹ ① ② ③ ④ ⑤ ⑥ ⑦ ⑧ ⑨ ⑩

caffeine ⟹ ① ② ③ ④ ⑤ ⑥ ⑦ ⑧ ⑨ ⑩

alcohol ⟹ ① ② ③ ④ ⑤ ⑥ ⑦ ⑧ ⑨ ⑩

HORMONES

☐ Menstruating ☐ Menopause ☐ PMS   ☐ N/A | other

COMPUTER USE / READING

☐ None   ☐ Some   ☐ A lot   Total time: [   ]

☐ Sitting   ☐ Standing   ☐ Mixture   Breaks every: [   ]

PHYSICAL ACTIVITY

☐ None   ☐ Minimal   ☐ Some   ☐ Sweatin'   ☐ I'm beat

DETAILS: _____

RELIEF MEASURES

☐ Medication   ☐ Massage   ☐ Sleep   ☐ Exercise

☐ Water   ☐ Cold/Ice   ☐ Heat/Bath   ☐ Other

DETAILS: _____

DID IT WORK? ☐ Nope   ☐ A bit   ☐ Mostly   ☐ 100%

Notes

Date: _____

START:	END:	DURATION:

| MIGRAINE | CLUSTER | SINUS | TMJ | TENSION |

PAIN LEVEL

1	2	3	4	5	6	7	8	9	10

Not too bad. *Well, I'm not enjoying this.* *Holy shit, make it stop!*

DETAILED DESCRIPTION

☐ Constant ☐ Squeezing ☐ Throbbing ☐ Pounding
☐ Dull aching ☐ Burning ☐ Sharp ☐ Debilitating

Other:_____

ONSET

☐ Slow ☐ Average ☐ Rapid ☐ Sudden

WHERE DOES IT HURT, EXACTLY?

OTHER SYMPTOMS

☐ Lightheaded ☐ Dizziness ☐ Confusion
☐ Light sensitivity ☐ Sound sensitivity ☐ Auras
☐ Muscle stiffness ☐ Muscle burning ☐ Muscle aches

HOW ARE YOU FEELING OVERALL?   Feeling sick?

Mood	① ② ③ ④ ⑤ ⑥ ⑦ ⑧ ⑨ ⑩	☐ Nope!
Energy levels	① ② ③ ④ ⑤ ⑥ ⑦ ⑧ ⑨ ⑩	☐ Yes...
Mental clarity	① ② ③ ④ ⑤ ⑥ ⑦ ⑧ ⑨ ⑩	

☐ Nausea ☐ Diarrhea ☐ Vomiting ☐ Sore throat
☐ Congestion ☐ Coughing ☐ Chills ☐ Fever

Other symptoms: _____

LAST NIGHT'S SLEEP

Hours of Sleep: _____   Sleep Quality: ① ② ③ ④ ⑤

WEATHER

☐ Hot   ☐ Mild   ☐ Cold   BM Pressure: _____

☐ Dry   ☐ Humid   ☐ Wet   Allergen Levels: _____

☐ Sunny   ☐ Cloudy

STRESS LEVELS

None	Low	Medium	High	Max	@$#%!

FOOD / DRINKS + NON-RELIEF MEDICATION / SUPPLEMENTS

item / meal	time	meds / supplements	dose	time

How many drinks?

water	➡	① ② ③ ④ ⑤ ⑥ ⑦ ⑧ ⑨ ⑩
caffeine	➡	① ② ③ ④ ⑤ ⑥ ⑦ ⑧ ⑨ ⑩
alcohol	➡	① ② ③ ④ ⑤ ⑥ ⑦ ⑧ ⑨ ⑩

HORMONES

☐ Menstruating   ☐ Menopause   ☐ PMS   ☐ N/A | other

COMPUTER USE / READING

☐ None   ☐ Some   ☐ A lot   Total time: [____]

☐ Sitting   ☐ Standing   ☐ Mixture   Breaks every: [____]

PHYSICAL ACTIVITY

☐ None   ☐ Minimal   ☐ Some   ☐ Sweatin'   ☐ I'm beat

DETAILS: _____

RELIEF MEASURES

☐ Medication   ☐ Massage   ☐ Sleep   ☐ Exercise

☐ Water   ☐ Cold/Ice   ☐ Heat/Bath   ☐ Other

DETAILS: _____

DID IT WORK?   ☐ Nope   ☐ A bit   ☐ Mostly   ☐ 100%

Notes

Date:_____

START:	END:	DURATION:

MIGRAINE	CLUSTER	SINUS	TMJ	TENSION

PAIN LEVEL

1	2	3	4	5	6	7	8	9	10

Not too bad.   *Well, I'm not enjoying this.*   *Holy shit, make it stop!*

DETAILED DESCRIPTION

☐ Constant   ☐ Squeezing   ☐ Throbbing   ☐ Pounding
☐ Dull aching ☐ Burning   ☐ Sharp   ☐ Debilitating

Other:_____

ONSET

☐ Slow   ☐ Average   ☐ Rapid   ☐ Sudden

WHERE DOES IT HURT, EXACTLY?

OTHER SYMPTOMS

☐ Lightheaded   ☐ Dizziness   ☐ Confusion
☐ Light sensitivity ☐ Sound sensitivity   ☐ Auras
☐ Muscle stiffness ☐ Muscle burning   ☐ Muscle aches

HOW ARE YOU FEELING OVERALL?

Feeling sick?

Mood	① ② ③ ④ ⑤ ⑥ ⑦ ⑧ ⑨ ⑩	☐ Nope!
Energy levels	① ② ③ ④ ⑤ ⑥ ⑦ ⑧ ⑨ ⑩	☐ Yes...
Mental clarity	① ② ③ ④ ⑤ ⑥ ⑦ ⑧ ⑨ ⑩	

☐ Nausea   ☐ Diarrhea   ☐ Vomiting   ☐ Sore throat
☐ Congestion   ☐ Coughing   ☐ Chills   ☐ Fever

Other symptoms:_____

LAST NIGHT'S SLEEP

Hours of Sleep: _____   Sleep Quality: ① ② ③ ④ ⑤

WEATHER

☐ Hot   ☐ Mild   ☐ Cold   BM Pressure: _____

☐ Dry   ☐ Humid   ☐ Wet   Allergen Levels: _____

☐ Sunny   ☐ Cloudy

STRESS LEVELS

None	Low	Medium	High	Max	@$#%!

FOOD / DRINKS + NON-RELIEF MEDICATION / SUPPLEMENTS

item / meal	time	meds / supplements	dose	time

How many drinks?

water   → ① ② ③ ④ ⑤ ⑥ ⑦ ⑧ ⑨ ⑩

caffeine   → ① ② ③ ④ ⑤ ⑥ ⑦ ⑧ ⑨ ⑩

alcohol   → ① ② ③ ④ ⑤ ⑥ ⑦ ⑧ ⑨ ⑩

HORMONES

☐ Menstruating   ☐ Menopause   ☐ PMS   ☐ N/A | other

COMPUTER USE / READING

☐ None   ☐ Some   ☐ A lot   Total time: [   ]

☐ Sitting   ☐ Standing   ☐ Mixture   Breaks every: [   ]

PHYSICAL ACTIVITY

☐ None   ☐ Minimal   ☐ Some   ☐ Sweatin'   ☐ I'm beat

DETAILS: _____

RELIEF MEASURES

☐ Medication   ☐ Massage   ☐ Sleep   ☐ Exercise

☐ Water   ☐ Cold/Ice   ☐ Heat/Bath   ☐ Other

DETAILS: _____

DID IT WORK?   ☐ Nope   ☐ A bit   ☐ Mostly   ☐ 100%

Notes

Date:_____

START:	END:	DURATION:

MIGRAINE	CLUSTER	SINUS	TMJ	TENSION

PAIN LEVEL

1	2	3	4	5	6	7	8	9	10

Not too bad.   *Well, I'm not enjoying this.*   *Holy shit, make it stop!*

DETAILED DESCRIPTION

☐ Constant   ☐ Squeezing   ☐ Throbbing   ☐ Pounding
☐ Dull aching   ☐ Burning   ☐ Sharp   ☐ Debilitating

Other:_____

ONSET

☐ Slow   ☐ Average   ☐ Rapid   ☐ Sudden

WHERE DOES IT HURT, EXACTLY?

OTHER SYMPTOMS

☐ Lightheaded   ☐ Dizziness   ☐ Confusion
☐ Light sensitivity   ☐ Sound sensitivity   ☐ Auras
☐ Muscle stiffness   ☐ Muscle burning   ☐ Muscle aches

HOW ARE YOU FEELING OVERALL?   Feeling sick?

Mood	① ② ③ ④ ⑤ ⑥ ⑦ ⑧ ⑨ ⑩	☐ Nope!
Energy levels	① ② ③ ④ ⑤ ⑥ ⑦ ⑧ ⑨ ⑩	☐ Yes...
Mental clarity	① ② ③ ④ ⑤ ⑥ ⑦ ⑧ ⑨ ⑩	

☐ Nausea   ☐ Diarrhea   ☐ Vomiting   ☐ Sore throat
☐ Congestion   ☐ Coughing   ☐ Chills   ☐ Fever

Other symptoms:_____

LAST NIGHT'S SLEEP

Hours of Sleep: _____   Sleep Quality: ① ② ③ ④ ⑤

WEATHER

☐ Hot   ☐ Mild   ☐ Cold   BM Pressure: _____

☐ Dry   ☐ Humid   ☐ Wet   Allergen Levels: _____

☐ Sunny   ☐ Cloudy

STRESS LEVELS

None	Low	Medium	High	Max	@$#%!

FOOD / DRINKS + NON-RELIEF MEDICATION / SUPPLEMENTS

item / meal	time	meds / supplements	dose	time

How many drinks?

water   → ① ② ③ ④ ⑤ ⑥ ⑦ ⑧ ⑨ ⑩

caffeine → ① ② ③ ④ ⑤ ⑥ ⑦ ⑧ ⑨ ⑩

alcohol → ① ② ③ ④ ⑤ ⑥ ⑦ ⑧ ⑨ ⑩

HORMONES

☐ Menstruating   ☐ Menopause   ☐ PMS   ☐ N/A | other

COMPUTER USE / READING

☐ None   ☐ Some   ☐ A lot   Total time: [   ]

☐ Sitting   ☐ Standing   ☐ Mixture   Breaks every: [   ]

PHYSICAL ACTIVITY

☐ None   ☐ Minimal   ☐ Some   ☐ Sweatin'   ☐ I'm beat

DETAILS: _____

RELIEF MEASURES

☐ Medication   ☐ Massage   ☐ Sleep   ☐ Exercise

☐ Water   ☐ Cold/Ice   ☐ Heat/Bath   ☐ Other

DETAILS: _____

DID IT WORK?   ☐ Nope   ☐ A bit   ☐ Mostly   ☐ 100%

Notes

Date:_____

START:	END:	DURATION:

MIGRAINE	CLUSTER	SINUS	TMJ	TENSION

PAIN LEVEL

1	2	3	4	5	6	7	8	9	10

Not too bad.   *Well, I'm not enjoying this.*   *Holy shit, make it stop!*

DETAILED DESCRIPTION

☐ Constant   ☐ Squeezing   ☐ Throbbing   ☐ Pounding
☐ Dull aching   ☐ Burning   ☐ Sharp   ☐ Debilitating

Other:_____

ONSET

☐ Slow   ☐ Average   ☐ Rapid   ☐ Sudden

WHERE DOES IT HURT, EXACTLY?

OTHER SYMPTOMS

☐ Lightheaded   ☐ Dizziness   ☐ Confusion
☐ Light sensitivity   ☐ Sound sensitivity   ☐ Auras
☐ Muscle stiffness   ☐ Muscle burning   ☐ Muscle aches

HOW ARE YOU FEELING OVERALL?   Feeling sick?

Mood	① ② ③ ④ ⑤ ⑥ ⑦ ⑧ ⑨ ⑩	☐ Nope!
Energy levels	① ② ③ ④ ⑤ ⑥ ⑦ ⑧ ⑨ ⑩	☐ Yes...
Mental clarity	① ② ③ ④ ⑤ ⑥ ⑦ ⑧ ⑨ ⑩	

☐ Nausea   ☐ Diarrhea   ☐ Vomiting   ☐ Sore throat
☐ Congestion   ☐ Coughing   ☐ Chills   ☐ Fever

Other symptoms: _____

LAST NIGHT'S SLEEP

Hours of Sleep: _____   Sleep Quality: ① ② ③ ④ ⑤

WEATHER

☐ Hot   ☐ Mild   ☐ Cold   BM Pressure: _____
☐ Dry   ☐ Humid   ☐ Wet   Allergen Levels: _____
☐ Sunny   ☐ Cloudy

STRESS LEVELS

None	Low	Medium	High	Max	@$#%!

FOOD / DRINKS + NON-RELIEF MEDICATION / SUPPLEMENTS

item / meal	time	meds / supplements	dose	time

How many drinks?

water	→	① ② ③ ④ ⑤ ⑥ ⑦ ⑧ ⑨ ⑩
caffeine	→	① ② ③ ④ ⑤ ⑥ ⑦ ⑧ ⑨ ⑩
alcohol	→	① ② ③ ④ ⑤ ⑥ ⑦ ⑧ ⑨ ⑩

HORMONES

☐ Menstruating   ☐ Menopause   ☐ PMS   ☐ N/A | other

COMPUTER USE / READING

☐ None   ☐ Some   ☐ A lot   Total time: [____]
☐ Sitting   ☐ Standing   ☐ Mixture   Breaks every: [____]

PHYSICAL ACTIVITY

☐ None   ☐ Minimal   ☐ Some   ☐ Sweatin'   ☐ I'm beat
DETAILS: _____

RELIEF MEASURES

☐ Medication   ☐ Massage   ☐ Sleep   ☐ Exercise
☐ Water   ☐ Cold/Ice   ☐ Heat/Bath   ☐ Other
DETAILS: _____

DID IT WORK?   ☐ Nope   ☐ A bit   ☐ Mostly   ☐ 100%

Notes

Date:_____

START:	END:	DURATION:

| MIGRAINE | CLUSTER | SINUS | TMJ | TENSION |

PAIN LEVEL

1	2	3	4	5	6	7	8	9	10

Not too bad.   *Well, I'm not enjoying this.*   *Holy shit, make it stop!*

DETAILED DESCRIPTION

☐ Constant   ☐ Squeezing   ☐ Throbbing   ☐ Pounding
☐ Dull aching   ☐ Burning   ☐ Sharp   ☐ Debilitating

Other:_____

ONSET

☐ Slow   ☐ Average   ☐ Rapid   ☐ Sudden

WHERE DOES IT HURT, EXACTLY?

OTHER SYMPTOMS

☐ Lightheaded   ☐ Dizziness   ☐ Confusion
☐ Light sensitivity   ☐ Sound sensitivity   ☐ Auras
☐ Muscle stiffness   ☐ Muscle burning   ☐ Muscle aches

HOW ARE YOU FEELING OVERALL?

Feeling sick?

Mood ① ② ③ ④ ⑤ ⑥ ⑦ ⑧ ⑨ ⑩   ☐ Nope!

Energy levels ① ② ③ ④ ⑤ ⑥ ⑦ ⑧ ⑨ ⑩   ☐ Yes...

Mental clarity ① ② ③ ④ ⑤ ⑥ ⑦ ⑧ ⑨ ⑩

☐ Nausea   ☐ Diarrhea   ☐ Vomiting   ☐ Sore throat
☐ Congestion   ☐ Coughing   ☐ Chills   ☐ Fever

Other symptoms: _____

LAST NIGHT'S SLEEP

Hours of Sleep: _____   Sleep Quality: ① ② ③ ④ ⑤

WEATHER

☐ Hot   ☐ Mild   ☐ Cold   BM Pressure: _____

☐ Dry   ☐ Humid   ☐ Wet   Allergen Levels: _____

☐ Sunny   ☐ Cloudy

STRESS LEVELS

| None | Low | Medium | High | Max | @$#%! |

FOOD / DRINKS + NON-RELIEF MEDICATION / SUPPLEMENTS

item / meal	time	meds / supplements	dose	time

How many drinks?

water	→	① ② ③ ④ ⑤ ⑥ ⑦ ⑧ ⑨ ⑩
caffeine	→	① ② ③ ④ ⑤ ⑥ ⑦ ⑧ ⑨ ⑩
alcohol	→	① ② ③ ④ ⑤ ⑥ ⑦ ⑧ ⑨ ⑩

HORMONES

☐ Menstruating   ☐ Menopause   ☐ PMS   ☐ N/A | other

COMPUTER USE / READING

☐ None   ☐ Some   ☐ A lot   Total time: [_____]

☐ Sitting   ☐ Standing   ☐ Mixture   Breaks every: [_____]

PHYSICAL ACTIVITY

☐ None   ☐ Minimal   ☐ Some   ☐ Sweatin'   ☐ I'm beat

DETAILS: _____

RELIEF MEASURES

☐ Medication   ☐ Massage   ☐ Sleep   ☐ Exercise

☐ Water   ☐ Cold/Ice   ☐ Heat/Bath   ☐ Other

DETAILS: _____

DID IT WORK?   ☐ Nope   ☐ A bit   ☐ Mostly   ☐ 100%

Notes

Date:_____

START:	END:	DURATION:

MIGRAINE	CLUSTER	SINUS	TMJ	TENSION

PAIN LEVEL

1	2	3	4	5	6	7	8	9	10

Not too bad.　　　*Well, I'm not enjoying this.*　　　*Holy shit, make it stop!*

DETAILED DESCRIPTION

☐ Constant ☐ Squeezing ☐ Throbbing ☐ Pounding
☐ Dull aching ☐ Burning ☐ Sharp ☐ Debilitating

Other:_____

ONSET

☐ Slow ☐ Average ☐ Rapid ☐ Sudden

WHERE DOES IT HURT, EXACTLY?

OTHER SYMPTOMS

☐ Lightheaded ☐ Dizziness ☐ Confusion
☐ Light sensitivity ☐ Sound sensitivity ☐ Auras
☐ Muscle stiffness ☐ Muscle burning ☐ Muscle aches

HOW ARE YOU FEELING OVERALL?

Feeling sick?

Mood	① ② ③ ④ ⑤ ⑥ ⑦ ⑧ ⑨ ⑩	☐ Nope!
Energy levels	① ② ③ ④ ⑤ ⑥ ⑦ ⑧ ⑨ ⑩	☐ Yes...
Mental clarity	① ② ③ ④ ⑤ ⑥ ⑦ ⑧ ⑨ ⑩	

☐ Nausea ☐ Diarrhea ☐ Vomiting ☐ Sore throat
☐ Congestion ☐ Coughing ☐ Chills ☐ Fever

Other symptoms: _____

LAST NIGHT'S SLEEP

Hours of Sleep: _____   Sleep Quality: ① ② ③ ④ ⑤

WEATHER

☐ Hot ☐ Mild ☐ Cold   BM Pressure: _____

☐ Dry ☐ Humid ☐ Wet   Allergen Levels: _____

☐ Sunny ☐ Cloudy

STRESS LEVELS

None	Low	Medium	High	Max	@$#%!

FOOD / DRINKS + NON-RELIEF MEDICATION / SUPPLEMENTS

item / meal	time	meds / supplements	dose	time

How many drinks?

water → ① ② ③ ④ ⑤ ⑥ ⑦ ⑧ ⑨ ⑩

caffeine → ① ② ③ ④ ⑤ ⑥ ⑦ ⑧ ⑨ ⑩

alcohol → ① ② ③ ④ ⑤ ⑥ ⑦ ⑧ ⑨ ⑩

HORMONES

☐ Menstruating ☐ Menopause ☐ PMS   ☐ N/A | other

COMPUTER USE / READING

☐ None ☐ Some ☐ A lot   Total time: [   ]

☐ Sitting ☐ Standing ☐ Mixture   Breaks every: [   ]

PHYSICAL ACTIVITY

☐ None ☐ Minimal ☐ Some   ☐ Sweatin' ☐ I'm beat

DETAILS: _____

RELIEF MEASURES

☐ Medication ☐ Massage ☐ Sleep ☐ Exercise

☐ Water ☐ Cold/Ice ☐ Heat/Bath ☐ Other

DETAILS: _____

DID IT WORK? ☐ Nope ☐ A bit ☐ Mostly ☐ 100%

Notes

Date:_____

START:	END:	DURATION:

MIGRAINE	CLUSTER	SINUS	TMJ	TENSION

PAIN LEVEL

1	2	3	4	5	6	7	8	9	10

Not too bad. *Well, I'm not enjoying this.* *Holy shit, make it stop!*

DETAILED DESCRIPTION

☐ Constant   ☐ Squeezing   ☐ Throbbing   ☐ Pounding
☐ Dull aching   ☐ Burning   ☐ Sharp   ☐ Debilitating

Other:_____

ONSET

☐ Slow   ☐ Average   ☐ Rapid   ☐ Sudden

WHERE DOES IT HURT, EXACTLY?

OTHER SYMPTOMS

☐ Lightheaded   ☐ Dizziness   ☐ Confusion
☐ Light sensitivity   ☐ Sound sensitivity   ☐ Auras
☐ Muscle stiffness   ☐ Muscle burning   ☐ Muscle aches

HOW ARE YOU FEELING OVERALL?

Feeling sick?

Mood	① ② ③ ④ ⑤ ⑥ ⑦ ⑧ ⑨ ⑩	☐ Nope!
Energy levels	① ② ③ ④ ⑤ ⑥ ⑦ ⑧ ⑨ ⑩	☐ Yes…
Mental clarity	① ② ③ ④ ⑤ ⑥ ⑦ ⑧ ⑨ ⑩	

☐ Nausea   ☐ Diarrhea   ☐ Vomiting   ☐ Sore throat
☐ Congestion   ☐ Coughing   ☐ Chills   ☐ Fever

Other symptoms: _____

LAST NIGHT'S SLEEP

Hours of Sleep: _____   Sleep Quality: ① ② ③ ④ ⑤

WEATHER

☐ Hot   ☐ Mild   ☐ Cold   BM Pressure: _____

☐ Dry   ☐ Humid   ☐ Wet   Allergen Levels: _____

☐ Sunny   ☐ Cloudy

STRESS LEVELS

None	Low	Medium	High	Max	@$#%!

FOOD / DRINKS + NON-RELIEF MEDICATION / SUPPLEMENTS

item / meal	time	meds / supplements	dose	time

How many drinks?

water ⟶ ① ② ③ ④ ⑤ ⑥ ⑦ ⑧ ⑨ ⑩

caffeine ⟶ ① ② ③ ④ ⑤ ⑥ ⑦ ⑧ ⑨ ⑩

alcohol ⟶ ① ② ③ ④ ⑤ ⑥ ⑦ ⑧ ⑨ ⑩

HORMONES

☐ Menstruating   ☐ Menopause   ☐ PMS   ☐ N/A | other

COMPUTER USE / READING

☐ None   ☐ Some   ☐ A lot   Total time: [   ]

☐ Sitting   ☐ Standing   ☐ Mixture   Breaks every: [   ]

PHYSICAL ACTIVITY

☐ None   ☐ Minimal   ☐ Some   ☐ Sweatin'   ☐ I'm beat

DETAILS: _____

RELIEF MEASURES

☐ Medication   ☐ Massage   ☐ Sleep   ☐ Exercise

☐ Water   ☐ Cold/Ice   ☐ Heat/Bath   ☐ Other

DETAILS: _____

DID IT WORK?   ☐ Nope   ☐ A bit   ☐ Mostly   ☐ 100%

Notes

Date:_____

START:	END:	DURATION:

| MIGRAINE | CLUSTER | SINUS | TMJ | TENSION |

PAIN LEVEL

1	2	3	4	5	6	7	8	9	10

Not too bad.   *Well, I'm not enjoying this.*   *Holy shit, make it stop!*

DETAILED DESCRIPTION

☐ Constant   ☐ Squeezing   ☐ Throbbing   ☐ Pounding
☐ Dull aching   ☐ Burning   ☐ Sharp   ☐ Debilitating

Other:_____

ONSET

☐ Slow   ☐ Average   ☐ Rapid   ☐ Sudden

WHERE DOES IT HURT, EXACTLY?

OTHER SYMPTOMS

☐ Lightheaded   ☐ Dizziness   ☐ Confusion
☐ Light sensitivity   ☐ Sound sensitivity   ☐ Auras
☐ Muscle stiffness   ☐ Muscle burning   ☐ Muscle aches

HOW ARE YOU FEELING OVERALL?

Feeling sick?

Mood   ① ② ③ ④ ⑤ ⑥ ⑦ ⑧ ⑨ ⑩   ☐ Nope!

Energy levels   ① ② ③ ④ ⑤ ⑥ ⑦ ⑧ ⑨ ⑩   ☐ Yes...

Mental clarity   ① ② ③ ④ ⑤ ⑥ ⑦ ⑧ ⑨ ⑩

| ☐ Nausea | ☐ Diarrhea | ☐ Vomiting | ☐ Sore throat |
| ☐ Congestion | ☐ Coughing | ☐ Chills | ☐ Fever |

Other symptoms: _____

LAST NIGHT'S SLEEP

Hours of Sleep: _____   Sleep Quality: ① ② ③ ④ ⑤

WEATHER

☐ Hot   ☐ Mild   ☐ Cold   BM Pressure: _____

☐ Dry   ☐ Humid   ☐ Wet   Allergen Levels: _____

☐ Sunny   ☐ Cloudy

STRESS LEVELS

None	Low	Medium	High	Max	@$#%!

FOOD / DRINKS + NON-RELIEF MEDICATION / SUPPLEMENTS

item / meal	time	meds / supplements	dose	time
		How many drinks?		

water ⟹ ① ② ③ ④ ⑤ ⑥ ⑦ ⑧ ⑨ ⑩

caffeine ⟹ ① ② ③ ④ ⑤ ⑥ ⑦ ⑧ ⑨ ⑩

alcohol ⟹ ① ② ③ ④ ⑤ ⑥ ⑦ ⑧ ⑨ ⑩

HORMONES

☐ Menstruating   ☐ Menopause   ☐ PMS   ☐ N/A | other

COMPUTER USE / READING

☐ None   ☐ Some   ☐ A lot   Total time: [____]

☐ Sitting   ☐ Standing   ☐ Mixture   Breaks every: [____]

PHYSICAL ACTIVITY

☐ None   ☐ Minimal   ☐ Some   ☐ Sweatin'   ☐ I'm beat

DETAILS: _____

RELIEF MEASURES

☐ Medication   ☐ Massage   ☐ Sleep   ☐ Exercise

☐ Water   ☐ Cold/Ice   ☐ Heat/Bath   ☐ Other

DETAILS: _____

DID IT WORK?   ☐ Nope   ☐ A bit   ☐ Mostly   ☐ 100%

Notes

Date:_____

START:	END:	DURATION:

MIGRAINE	CLUSTER	SINUS	TMJ	TENSION

PAIN LEVEL

1	2	3	4	5	6	7	8	9	10

Not too bad.   *Well, I'm not enjoying this.*   *Holy shit, make it stop!*

DETAILED DESCRIPTION

☐ Constant   ☐ Squeezing   ☐ Throbbing   ☐ Pounding
☐ Dull aching   ☐ Burning   ☐ Sharp   ☐ Debilitating

Other:_____

ONSET

☐ Slow   ☐ Average   ☐ Rapid   ☐ Sudden

WHERE DOES IT HURT, EXACTLY?

OTHER SYMPTOMS

☐ Lightheaded   ☐ Dizziness   ☐ Confusion
☐ Light sensitivity   ☐ Sound sensitivity   ☐ Auras
☐ Muscle stiffness   ☐ Muscle burning   ☐ Muscle aches

HOW ARE YOU FEELING OVERALL?

Feeling sick?

Mood	① ② ③ ④ ⑤ ⑥ ⑦ ⑧ ⑨ ⑩	☐ Nope!
Energy levels	① ② ③ ④ ⑤ ⑥ ⑦ ⑧ ⑨ ⑩	☐ Yes...
Mental clarity	① ② ③ ④ ⑤ ⑥ ⑦ ⑧ ⑨ ⑩	

☐ Nausea   ☐ Diarrhea   ☐ Vomiting   ☐ Sore throat
☐ Congestion   ☐ Coughing   ☐ Chills   ☐ Fever

Other symptoms: _____

LAST NIGHT'S SLEEP

Hours of Sleep: _____   Sleep Quality: ① ② ③ ④ ⑤

WEATHER

☐ Hot   ☐ Mild   ☐ Cold   BM Pressure: _____

☐ Dry   ☐ Humid   ☐ Wet   Allergen Levels: _____

☐ Sunny   ☐ Cloudy

STRESS LEVELS

None	Low	Medium	High	Max	@$#%!

FOOD / DRINKS + NON-RELIEF MEDICATION / SUPPLEMENTS

item / meal	time	meds / supplements	dose	time

How many drinks?

water   → ① ② ③ ④ ⑤ ⑥ ⑦ ⑧ ⑨ ⑩

caffeine → ① ② ③ ④ ⑤ ⑥ ⑦ ⑧ ⑨ ⑩

alcohol → ① ② ③ ④ ⑤ ⑥ ⑦ ⑧ ⑨ ⑩

HORMONES

☐ Menstruating   ☐ Menopause   ☐ PMS   ☐ N/A | other

COMPUTER USE / READING

☐ None   ☐ Some   ☐ A lot   Total time: _____

☐ Sitting   ☐ Standing   ☐ Mixture   Breaks every: _____

PHYSICAL ACTIVITY

☐ None   ☐ Minimal   ☐ Some   ☐ Sweatin'   ☐ I'm beat

DETAILS: _____

RELIEF MEASURES

☐ Medication   ☐ Massage   ☐ Sleep   ☐ Exercise

☐ Water   ☐ Cold/Ice   ☐ Heat/Bath   ☐ Other

DETAILS: _____

DID IT WORK?   ☐ Nope   ☐ A bit   ☐ Mostly   ☐ 100%

Notes

Date:_____

START: | **END:** | **DURATION:**

| MIGRAINE | CLUSTER | SINUS | TMJ | TENSION |

PAIN LEVEL

1	2	3	4	5	6	7	8	9	10

Not too bad.　　*Well, I'm not enjoying this.*　　*Holy shit, make it stop!*

DETAILED DESCRIPTION

☐ Constant ☐ Squeezing ☐ Throbbing ☐ Pounding
☐ Dull aching ☐ Burning ☐ Sharp ☐ Debilitating

Other:_____

ONSET

☐ Slow ☐ Average ☐ Rapid ☐ Sudden

WHERE DOES IT HURT, EXACTLY?

OTHER SYMPTOMS

☐ Lightheaded ☐ Dizziness ☐ Confusion
☐ Light sensitivity ☐ Sound sensitivity ☐ Auras
☐ Muscle stiffness ☐ Muscle burning ☐ Muscle aches

HOW ARE YOU FEELING OVERALL?

Feeling sick?

Mood ① ② ③ ④ ⑤ ⑥ ⑦ ⑧ ⑨ ⑩ ☐ Nope!

Energy levels ① ② ③ ④ ⑤ ⑥ ⑦ ⑧ ⑨ ⑩ ☐ Yes...

Mental clarity ① ② ③ ④ ⑤ ⑥ ⑦ ⑧ ⑨ ⑩

☐ Nausea ☐ Diarrhea ☐ Vomiting ☐ Sore throat
☐ Congestion ☐ Coughing ☐ Chills ☐ Fever

Other symptoms: _____

LAST NIGHT'S SLEEP

Hours of Sleep: _____ Sleep Quality: ① ② ③ ④ ⑤

WEATHER

☐ Hot   ☐ Mild   ☐ Cold   BM Pressure: _____

☐ Dry   ☐ Humid   ☐ Wet   Allergen Levels: _____

☐ Sunny   ☐ Cloudy

STRESS LEVELS

None	Low	Medium	High	Max	@$#%!

FOOD / DRINKS + NON-RELIEF MEDICATION / SUPPLEMENTS

item / meal	time	meds / supplements	dose	time

How many drinks? ⟶

water ⟹ ① ② ③ ④ ⑤ ⑥ ⑦ ⑧ ⑨ ⑩

caffeine ⟹ ① ② ③ ④ ⑤ ⑥ ⑦ ⑧ ⑨ ⑩

alcohol ⟹ ① ② ③ ④ ⑤ ⑥ ⑦ ⑧ ⑨ ⑩

HORMONES

☐ Menstruating   ☐ Menopause   ☐ PMS   ☐ N/A | other

COMPUTER USE / READING

☐ None   ☐ Some   ☐ A lot   Total time: _____

☐ Sitting   ☐ Standing   ☐ Mixture   Breaks every: _____

PHYSICAL ACTIVITY

☐ None   ☐ Minimal   ☐ Some   ☐ Sweatin'   ☐ I'm beat

DETAILS: _____

RELIEF MEASURES

☐ Medication   ☐ Massage   ☐ Sleep   ☐ Exercise

☐ Water   ☐ Cold/Ice   ☐ Heat/Bath   ☐ Other

DETAILS: _____

DID IT WORK?   ☐ Nope   ☐ A bit   ☐ Mostly   ☐ 100%

Notes

Date:_____

START:	END:	DURATION:

MIGRAINE	CLUSTER	SINUS	TMJ	TENSION

PAIN LEVEL

1	2	3	4	5	6	7	8	9	10

Not too bad.   *Well, I'm not enjoying this.*   *Holy shit, make it stop!*

DETAILED DESCRIPTION

☐ Constant   ☐ Squeezing   ☐ Throbbing   ☐ Pounding
☐ Dull aching   ☐ Burning   ☐ Sharp   ☐ Debilitating

Other:_____

ONSET

☐ Slow   ☐ Average   ☐ Rapid   ☐ Sudden

WHERE DOES IT HURT, EXACTLY?

OTHER SYMPTOMS

☐ Lightheaded   ☐ Dizziness   ☐ Confusion
☐ Light sensitivity   ☐ Sound sensitivity   ☐ Auras
☐ Muscle stiffness   ☐ Muscle burning   ☐ Muscle aches

HOW ARE YOU FEELING OVERALL?

Feeling sick?

Mood	① ② ③ ④ ⑤ ⑥ ⑦ ⑧ ⑨ ⑩	☐ Nope!
Energy levels	① ② ③ ④ ⑤ ⑥ ⑦ ⑧ ⑨ ⑩	☐ Yes...
Mental clarity	① ② ③ ④ ⑤ ⑥ ⑦ ⑧ ⑨ ⑩	

☐ Nausea   ☐ Diarrhea   ☐ Vomiting   ☐ Sore throat
☐ Congestion   ☐ Coughing   ☐ Chills   ☐ Fever

Other symptoms: _____

LAST NIGHT'S SLEEP

Hours of Sleep: _____   Sleep Quality: ① ② ③ ④ ⑤

WEATHER

☐ Hot   ☐ Mild   ☐ Cold   BM Pressure: _____

☐ Dry   ☐ Humid   ☐ Wet   Allergen Levels: _____

☐ Sunny   ☐ Cloudy

STRESS LEVELS

None	Low	Medium	High	Max	@$#%!

FOOD / DRINKS + NON-RELIEF MEDICATION / SUPPLEMENTS

item / meal	time	meds / supplements	dose	time
		How many drinks?		

water ➡ ① ② ③ ④ ⑤ ⑥ ⑦ ⑧ ⑨ ⑩

caffeine ➡ ① ② ③ ④ ⑤ ⑥ ⑦ ⑧ ⑨ ⑩

alcohol ➡ ① ② ③ ④ ⑤ ⑥ ⑦ ⑧ ⑨ ⑩

HORMONES

☐ Menstruating   ☐ Menopause   ☐ PMS   ☐ N/A | other

COMPUTER USE / READING

☐ None   ☐ Some   ☐ A lot   Total time: [____]

☐ Sitting   ☐ Standing   ☐ Mixture   Breaks every: [____]

PHYSICAL ACTIVITY

☐ None   ☐ Minimal   ☐ Some   ☐ Sweatin'   ☐ I'm beat

DETAILS: _____

RELIEF MEASURES

☐ Medication   ☐ Massage   ☐ Sleep   ☐ Exercise

☐ Water   ☐ Cold/Ice   ☐ Heat/Bath   ☐ Other

DETAILS: _____

DID IT WORK?   ☐ Nope   ☐ A bit   ☐ Mostly   ☐ 100%

Notes

Date:_____

START:	END:	DURATION:

MIGRAINE CLUSTER SINUS TMJ TENSION

PAIN LEVEL

1	2	3	4	5	6	7	8	9	10

Not too bad.   *Well, I'm not enjoying this.*   *Holy shit, make it stop!*

DETAILED DESCRIPTION

☐ Constant   ☐ Squeezing   ☐ Throbbing   ☐ Pounding
☐ Dull aching   ☐ Burning   ☐ Sharp   ☐ Debilitating

Other:_____

ONSET

☐ Slow   ☐ Average   ☐ Rapid   ☐ Sudden

WHERE DOES IT HURT, EXACTLY?

OTHER SYMPTOMS

☐ Lightheaded   ☐ Dizziness   ☐ Confusion
☐ Light sensitivity   ☐ Sound sensitivity   ☐ Auras
☐ Muscle stiffness   ☐ Muscle burning   ☐ Muscle aches

HOW ARE YOU FEELING OVERALL?   Feeling sick?

Mood	① ② ③ ④ ⑤ ⑥ ⑦ ⑧ ⑨ ⑩	☐ Nope!
Energy levels	① ② ③ ④ ⑤ ⑥ ⑦ ⑧ ⑨ ⑩	☐ Yes...
Mental clarity	① ② ③ ④ ⑤ ⑥ ⑦ ⑧ ⑨ ⑩	

☐ Nausea   ☐ Diarrhea   ☐ Vomiting   ☐ Sore throat
☐ Congestion   ☐ Coughing   ☐ Chills   ☐ Fever

Other symptoms: _____

LAST NIGHT'S SLEEP

Hours of Sleep: _____   Sleep Quality: ① ② ③ ④ ⑤

WEATHER

☐ Hot   ☐ Mild   ☐ Cold   BM Pressure: _____

☐ Dry   ☐ Humid   ☐ Wet   Allergen Levels: _____

☐ Sunny   ☐ Cloudy

STRESS LEVELS

None	Low	Medium	High	Max	@$#%!

FOOD / DRINKS + NON-RELIEF MEDICATION / SUPPLEMENTS

item / meal	time	meds / supplements	dose	time

How many drinks?

water   ① ② ③ ④ ⑤ ⑥ ⑦ ⑧ ⑨ ⑩

caffeine ① ② ③ ④ ⑤ ⑥ ⑦ ⑧ ⑨ ⑩

alcohol ① ② ③ ④ ⑤ ⑥ ⑦ ⑧ ⑨ ⑩

HORMONES

☐ Menstruating   ☐ Menopause   ☐ PMS   ☐ N/A | other

COMPUTER USE / READING

☐ None   ☐ Some   ☐ A lot   Total time: [   ]

☐ Sitting   ☐ Standing   ☐ Mixture   Breaks every: [   ]

PHYSICAL ACTIVITY

☐ None   ☐ Minimal   ☐ Some   ☐ Sweatin'   ☐ I'm beat

DETAILS: _____

RELIEF MEASURES

☐ Medication   ☐ Massage   ☐ Sleep   ☐ Exercise

☐ Water   ☐ Cold/Ice   ☐ Heat/Bath   ☐ Other

DETAILS: _____

DID IT WORK?   ☐ Nope   ☐ A bit   ☐ Mostly   ☐ 100%

Notes

Date:_____

START: [　　　]   END: [　　　]   DURATION: [　　　]

| MIGRAINE | CLUSTER | SINUS | TMJ | TENSION |

PAIN LEVEL

1	2	3	4	5	6	7	8	9	10

Not too bad.   *Well, I'm not enjoying this.*   *Holy shit, make it stop!*

DETAILED DESCRIPTION

☐ Constant ☐ Squeezing ☐ Throbbing ☐ Pounding
☐ Dull aching ☐ Burning ☐ Sharp ☐ Debilitating

Other:_____

ONSET

☐ Slow ☐ Average ☐ Rapid ☐ Sudden

WHERE DOES IT HURT, EXACTLY?

OTHER SYMPTOMS

☐ Lightheaded ☐ Dizziness ☐ Confusion
☐ Light sensitivity ☐ Sound sensitivity ☐ Auras
☐ Muscle stiffness ☐ Muscle burning ☐ Muscle aches

HOW ARE YOU FEELING OVERALL?

Feeling sick?

Mood	① ② ③ ④ ⑤ ⑥ ⑦ ⑧ ⑨ ⑩	☐ Nope!
Energy levels	① ② ③ ④ ⑤ ⑥ ⑦ ⑧ ⑨ ⑩	☐ Yes...
Mental clarity	① ② ③ ④ ⑤ ⑥ ⑦ ⑧ ⑨ ⑩	

☐ Nausea ☐ Diarrhea ☐ Vomiting ☐ Sore throat
☐ Congestion ☐ Coughing ☐ Chills ☐ Fever

Other symptoms: _____

LAST NIGHT'S SLEEP

Hours of Sleep: _____   Sleep Quality: ① ② ③ ④ ⑤

WEATHER

☐ Hot   ☐ Mild   ☐ Cold   BM Pressure: _____

☐ Dry   ☐ Humid   ☐ Wet   Allergen Levels: _____

☐ Sunny   ☐ Cloudy

STRESS LEVELS

None	Low	Medium	High	Max	@$#%!

FOOD / DRINKS + NON-RELIEF MEDICATION / SUPPLEMENTS

item / meal	time	meds / supplements	dose	time

How many drinks?

water   ① ② ③ ④ ⑤ ⑥ ⑦ ⑧ ⑨ ⑩

caffeine ① ② ③ ④ ⑤ ⑥ ⑦ ⑧ ⑨ ⑩

alcohol ① ② ③ ④ ⑤ ⑥ ⑦ ⑧ ⑨ ⑩

HORMONES

☐ Menstruating   ☐ Menopause   ☐ PMS   ☐ N/A | other

COMPUTER USE / READING

☐ None   ☐ Some   ☐ A lot   Total time: [   ]

☐ Sitting   ☐ Standing   ☐ Mixture   Breaks every: [   ]

PHYSICAL ACTIVITY

☐ None   ☐ Minimal   ☐ Some   ☐ Sweatin'   ☐ I'm beat

DETAILS: _____

RELIEF MEASURES

☐ Medication   ☐ Massage   ☐ Sleep   ☐ Exercise

☐ Water   ☐ Cold/Ice   ☐ Heat/Bath   ☐ Other

DETAILS: _____

DID IT WORK?   ☐ Nope   ☐ A bit   ☐ Mostly   ☐ 100%

Notes

Date:_____

| START: | END: | DURATION: |

| MIGRAINE | CLUSTER | SINUS | TMJ | TENSION |

PAIN LEVEL

| 1 | 2 | 3 | 4 | 5 | 6 | 7 | 8 | 9 | 10 |

Not too bad.   *Well, I'm not enjoying this.*   *Holy shit, make it stop!*

DETAILED DESCRIPTION

☐ Constant ☐ Squeezing ☐ Throbbing ☐ Pounding
☐ Dull aching ☐ Burning ☐ Sharp ☐ Debilitating

Other:_____

ONSET

☐ Slow ☐ Average ☐ Rapid ☐ Sudden

WHERE DOES IT HURT, EXACTLY?

OTHER SYMPTOMS

☐ Lightheaded ☐ Dizziness ☐ Confusion
☐ Light sensitivity ☐ Sound sensitivity ☐ Auras
☐ Muscle stiffness ☐ Muscle burning ☐ Muscle aches

HOW ARE YOU FEELING OVERALL?

Feeling sick?

Mood	① ② ③ ④ ⑤ ⑥ ⑦ ⑧ ⑨ ⑩	☐ Nope!
Energy levels	① ② ③ ④ ⑤ ⑥ ⑦ ⑧ ⑨ ⑩	☐ Yes...
Mental clarity	① ② ③ ④ ⑤ ⑥ ⑦ ⑧ ⑨ ⑩	

☐ Nausea ☐ Diarrhea ☐ Vomiting ☐ Sore throat
☐ Congestion ☐ Coughing ☐ Chills ☐ Fever

Other symptoms: _____

LAST NIGHT'S SLEEP

Hours of Sleep: _____   Sleep Quality: ① ② ③ ④ ⑤

WEATHER

☐ Hot   ☐ Mild   ☐ Cold   BM Pressure: _____

☐ Dry   ☐ Humid   ☐ Wet   Allergen Levels: _____

☐ Sunny   ☐ Cloudy

STRESS LEVELS

None	Low	Medium	High	Max	@$#%!

FOOD / DRINKS + NON-RELIEF MEDICATION / SUPPLEMENTS

item / meal	time	meds / supplements	dose	time

How many drinks?

water   ① ② ③ ④ ⑤ ⑥ ⑦ ⑧ ⑨ ⑩

caffeine ① ② ③ ④ ⑤ ⑥ ⑦ ⑧ ⑨ ⑩

alcohol ① ② ③ ④ ⑤ ⑥ ⑦ ⑧ ⑨ ⑩

HORMONES

☐ Menstruating   ☐ Menopause   ☐ PMS   ☐ N/A | other

COMPUTER USE / READING

☐ None   ☐ Some   ☐ A lot   Total time: [   ]

☐ Sitting   ☐ Standing   ☐ Mixture   Breaks every: [   ]

PHYSICAL ACTIVITY

☐ None   ☐ Minimal   ☐ Some   ☐ Sweatin'   ☐ I'm beat

DETAILS: _____

RELIEF MEASURES

☐ Medication   ☐ Massage   ☐ Sleep   ☐ Exercise

☐ Water   ☐ Cold/Ice   ☐ Heat/Bath   ☐ Other

DETAILS: _____

DID IT WORK?   ☐ Nope   ☐ A bit   ☐ Mostly   ☐ 100%

Notes

Date:_____

START:	END:	DURATION:

| MIGRAINE | CLUSTER | SINUS | TMJ | TENSION |

PAIN LEVEL

1	2	3	4	5	6	7	8	9	10

Not too bad.   *Well, I'm not enjoying this.*   *Holy shit, make it stop!*

DETAILED DESCRIPTION

☐ Constant   ☐ Squeezing   ☐ Throbbing   ☐ Pounding
☐ Dull aching   ☐ Burning   ☐ Sharp   ☐ Debilitating

Other:_____

ONSET

☐ Slow   ☐ Average   ☐ Rapid   ☐ Sudden

WHERE DOES IT HURT, EXACTLY?

OTHER SYMPTOMS

☐ Lightheaded   ☐ Dizziness   ☐ Confusion
☐ Light sensitivity   ☐ Sound sensitivity   ☐ Auras
☐ Muscle stiffness   ☐ Muscle burning   ☐ Muscle aches

HOW ARE YOU FEELING OVERALL?

Feeling sick?

Mood   ①②③④⑤⑥⑦⑧⑨⑩   ☐ Nope!
Energy levels   ①②③④⑤⑥⑦⑧⑨⑩   ☐ Yes...
Mental clarity   ①②③④⑤⑥⑦⑧⑨⑩

☐ Nausea   ☐ Diarrhea   ☐ Vomiting   ☐ Sore throat
☐ Congestion   ☐ Coughing   ☐ Chills   ☐ Fever

Other symptoms: _____

LAST NIGHT'S SLEEP
Hours of Sleep: _____   Sleep Quality: ① ② ③ ④ ⑤

WEATHER

☐ Hot   ☐ Mild   ☐ Cold   BM Pressure: _____
☐ Dry   ☐ Humid   ☐ Wet   Allergen Levels: _____
☐ Sunny   ☐ Cloudy

STRESS LEVELS

None	Low	Medium	High	Max	@$#%!

FOOD / DRINKS + NON-RELIEF MEDICATION / SUPPLEMENTS

item / meal	time	meds / supplements	dose	time

How many drinks?

water → ① ② ③ ④ ⑤ ⑥ ⑦ ⑧ ⑨ ⑩
caffeine → ① ② ③ ④ ⑤ ⑥ ⑦ ⑧ ⑨ ⑩
alcohol → ① ② ③ ④ ⑤ ⑥ ⑦ ⑧ ⑨ ⑩

HORMONES
☐ Menstruating ☐ Menopause ☐ PMS   ☐ N/A | other

COMPUTER USE / READING
☐ None   ☐ Some   ☐ A lot   Total time: [   ]
☐ Sitting   ☐ Standing   ☐ Mixture   Breaks every: [   ]

PHYSICAL ACTIVITY
☐ None   ☐ Minimal   ☐ Some   ☐ Sweatin'   ☐ I'm beat
DETAILS: _____

RELIEF MEASURES
☐ Medication ☐ Massage   ☐ Sleep   ☐ Exercise
☐ Water   ☐ Cold/Ice   ☐ Heat/Bath   ☐ Other
DETAILS: _____

DID IT WORK? ☐ Nope   ☐ A bit   ☐ Mostly   ☐ 100%

Notes

Date:_____

START:	END:	DURATION:

MIGRAINE   CLUSTER   SINUS   TMJ   TENSION

PAIN LEVEL

1	2	3	4	5	6	7	8	9	10

Not too bad.   *Well, I'm not enjoying this.*   *Holy shit, make it stop!*

DETAILED DESCRIPTION

☐ Constant   ☐ Squeezing   ☐ Throbbing   ☐ Pounding
☐ Dull aching   ☐ Burning   ☐ Sharp   ☐ Debilitating

Other:_____

ONSET

☐ Slow   ☐ Average   ☐ Rapid   ☐ Sudden

WHERE DOES IT HURT, EXACTLY?

OTHER SYMPTOMS

☐ Lightheaded   ☐ Dizziness   ☐ Confusion
☐ Light sensitivity   ☐ Sound sensitivity ☐ Auras
☐ Muscle stiffness   ☐ Muscle burning   ☐ Muscle aches

HOW ARE YOU FEELING OVERALL?   Feeling sick?

Mood	① ② ③ ④ ⑤ ⑥ ⑦ ⑧ ⑨ ⑩	☐ Nope!
Energy levels	① ② ③ ④ ⑤ ⑥ ⑦ ⑧ ⑨ ⑩	☐ Yes...
Mental clarity	① ② ③ ④ ⑤ ⑥ ⑦ ⑧ ⑨ ⑩	

☐ Nausea   ☐ Diarrhea   ☐ Vomiting   ☐ Sore throat
☐ Congestion   ☐ Coughing   ☐ Chills   ☐ Fever

Other symptoms: _____

LAST NIGHT'S SLEEP

Hours of Sleep: _____   Sleep Quality: ① ② ③ ④ ⑤

WEATHER

☐ Hot   ☐ Mild   ☐ Cold   BM Pressure: _____
☐ Dry   ☐ Humid   ☐ Wet   Allergen Levels: _____
☐ Sunny   ☐ Cloudy

STRESS LEVELS

| None | Low | Medium | High | Max | @$#%! |

FOOD / DRINKS + NON-RELIEF MEDICATION / SUPPLEMENTS

item / meal	time	meds / supplements	dose	time

How many drinks?

water ⟹ ① ② ③ ④ ⑤ ⑥ ⑦ ⑧ ⑨ ⑩
caffeine ⟹ ① ② ③ ④ ⑤ ⑥ ⑦ ⑧ ⑨ ⑩
alcohol ⟹ ① ② ③ ④ ⑤ ⑥ ⑦ ⑧ ⑨ ⑩

HORMONES

☐ Menstruating   ☐ Menopause   ☐ PMS   ☐ N/A | other

COMPUTER USE / READING

☐ None   ☐ Some   ☐ A lot   Total time: [   ]
☐ Sitting   ☐ Standing   ☐ Mixture   Breaks every: [   ]

PHYSICAL ACTIVITY

☐ None   ☐ Minimal   ☐ Some   ☐ Sweatin'   ☐ I'm beat
DETAILS: _____

RELIEF MEASURES

☐ Medication   ☐ Massage   ☐ Sleep   ☐ Exercise
☐ Water   ☐ Cold/Ice   ☐ Heat/Bath   ☐ Other
DETAILS: _____

DID IT WORK?   ☐ Nope   ☐ A bit   ☐ Mostly   ☐ 100%

Notes

Date:_____ M T W T F S S

START:	END:	DURATION:

MIGRAINE   CLUSTER   SINUS   TMJ   TENSION

PAIN LEVEL

1	2	3	4	5	6	7	8	9	10

Not too bad.   *Well, I'm not enjoying this.*   *Holy shit, make it stop!*

DETAILED DESCRIPTION

☐ Constant ☐ Squeezing ☐ Throbbing ☐ Pounding
☐ Dull aching ☐ Burning ☐ Sharp ☐ Debilitating

Other:_____

ONSET

☐ Slow ☐ Average ☐ Rapid ☐ Sudden

WHERE DOES IT HURT, EXACTLY?

OTHER SYMPTOMS

☐ Lightheaded ☐ Dizziness ☐ Confusion
☐ Light sensitivity ☐ Sound sensitivity ☐ Auras
☐ Muscle stiffness ☐ Muscle burning ☐ Muscle aches

HOW ARE YOU FEELING OVERALL?

Feeling sick?

Mood ① ② ③ ④ ⑤ ⑥ ⑦ ⑧ ⑨ ⑩   ☐ Nope!

Energy levels ① ② ③ ④ ⑤ ⑥ ⑦ ⑧ ⑨ ⑩   ☐ Yes...

Mental clarity ① ② ③ ④ ⑤ ⑥ ⑦ ⑧ ⑨ ⑩

☐ Nausea ☐ Diarrhea ☐ Vomiting ☐ Sore throat
☐ Congestion ☐ Coughing ☐ Chills ☐ Fever

Other symptoms: _____

LAST NIGHT'S SLEEP

Hours of Sleep: _____   Sleep Quality: ① ② ③ ④ ⑤

WEATHER

☐ Hot   ☐ Mild   ☐ Cold   BM Pressure: _____
☐ Dry   ☐ Humid   ☐ Wet   Allergen Levels: _____
☐ Sunny   ☐ Cloudy

STRESS LEVELS

| None | Low | Medium | High | Max | @$#%! |

FOOD / DRINKS + NON-RELIEF MEDICATION / SUPPLEMENTS

item / meal	time	meds / supplements	dose	time

How many drinks?

water	① ② ③ ④ ⑤ ⑥ ⑦ ⑧ ⑨ ⑩
caffeine	① ② ③ ④ ⑤ ⑥ ⑦ ⑧ ⑨ ⑩
alcohol	① ② ③ ④ ⑤ ⑥ ⑦ ⑧ ⑨ ⑩

HORMONES

☐ Menstruating   ☐ Menopause   ☐ PMS   ☐ N/A | other

COMPUTER USE / READING

☐ None   ☐ Some   ☐ A lot   Total time: [____]
☐ Sitting   ☐ Standing   ☐ Mixture   Breaks every: [____]

PHYSICAL ACTIVITY

☐ None   ☐ Minimal   ☐ Some   ☐ Sweatin'   ☐ I'm beat
DETAILS: _____

RELIEF MEASURES

☐ Medication   ☐ Massage   ☐ Sleep   ☐ Exercise
☐ Water   ☐ Cold/Ice   ☐ Heat/Bath   ☐ Other
DETAILS: _____

DID IT WORK?   ☐ Nope   ☐ A bit   ☐ Mostly   ☐ 100%

Notes

Date:_____

START:	END:	DURATION:

MIGRAINE   CLUSTER   SINUS   TMJ   TENSION

PAIN LEVEL

1	2	3	4	5	6	7	8	9	10

Not too bad.   *Well, I'm not enjoying this.*   *Holy shit, make it stop!*

DETAILED DESCRIPTION

☐ Constant   ☐ Squeezing   ☐ Throbbing   ☐ Pounding
☐ Dull aching   ☐ Burning   ☐ Sharp   ☐ Debilitating

Other:_____

ONSET

☐ Slow   ☐ Average   ☐ Rapid   ☐ Sudden

WHERE DOES IT HURT, EXACTLY?

OTHER SYMPTOMS

☐ Lightheaded   ☐ Dizziness   ☐ Confusion
☐ Light sensitivity ☐ Sound sensitivity ☐ Auras
☐ Muscle stiffness ☐ Muscle burning   ☐ Muscle aches

HOW ARE YOU FEELING OVERALL?   Feeling sick?

Mood	① ② ③ ④ ⑤ ⑥ ⑦ ⑧ ⑨ ⑩	☐ Nope!
Energy levels	① ② ③ ④ ⑤ ⑥ ⑦ ⑧ ⑨ ⑩	☐ Yes...
Mental clarity	① ② ③ ④ ⑤ ⑥ ⑦ ⑧ ⑨ ⑩	

☐ Nausea   ☐ Diarrhea   ☐ Vomiting   ☐ Sore throat
☐ Congestion   ☐ Coughing   ☐ Chills   ☐ Fever

Other symptoms: _____

LAST NIGHT'S SLEEP

Hours of Sleep: _____   Sleep Quality: ① ② ③ ④ ⑤

WEATHER

☐ Hot   ☐ Mild   ☐ Cold   BM Pressure: _____

☐ Dry   ☐ Humid   ☐ Wet   Allergen Levels: _____

☐ Sunny   ☐ Cloudy

STRESS LEVELS

None	Low	Medium	High	Max	@$#%!

FOOD / DRINKS + NON-RELIEF MEDICATION / SUPPLEMENTS

item / meal	time	meds / supplements	dose	time

How many drinks?

water   → ① ② ③ ④ ⑤ ⑥ ⑦ ⑧ ⑨ ⑩

caffeine → ① ② ③ ④ ⑤ ⑥ ⑦ ⑧ ⑨ ⑩

alcohol → ① ② ③ ④ ⑤ ⑥ ⑦ ⑧ ⑨ ⑩

HORMONES

☐ Menstruating   ☐ Menopause   ☐ PMS   ☐ N/A | other

COMPUTER USE / READING

☐ None   ☐ Some   ☐ A lot   Total time: [   ]

☐ Sitting   ☐ Standing   ☐ Mixture   Breaks every: [   ]

PHYSICAL ACTIVITY

☐ None   ☐ Minimal   ☐ Some   ☐ Sweatin'   ☐ I'm beat

DETAILS: _____

RELIEF MEASURES

☐ Medication   ☐ Massage   ☐ Sleep   ☐ Exercise

☐ Water   ☐ Cold/Ice   ☐ Heat/Bath   ☐ Other

DETAILS: _____

DID IT WORK?   ☐ Nope   ☐ A bit   ☐ Mostly   ☐ 100%

Notes

Date:_____

START:	END:	DURATION:

| MIGRAINE | CLUSTER | SINUS | TMJ | TENSION |

PAIN LEVEL

1	2	3	4	5	6	7	8	9	10

Not too bad.   *Well, I'm not enjoying this.*   *Holy shit, make it stop!*

DETAILED DESCRIPTION

☐ Constant   ☐ Squeezing   ☐ Throbbing   ☐ Pounding
☐ Dull aching   ☐ Burning   ☐ Sharp   ☐ Debilitating

Other:_____

ONSET

☐ Slow   ☐ Average   ☐ Rapid   ☐ Sudden

WHERE DOES IT HURT, EXACTLY?

OTHER SYMPTOMS

☐ Lightheaded   ☐ Dizziness   ☐ Confusion
☐ Light sensitivity   ☐ Sound sensitivity   ☐ Auras
☐ Muscle stiffness   ☐ Muscle burning   ☐ Muscle aches

HOW ARE YOU FEELING OVERALL?   Feeling sick?

Mood	① ② ③ ④ ⑤ ⑥ ⑦ ⑧ ⑨ ⑩	☐ Nope!
Energy levels	① ② ③ ④ ⑤ ⑥ ⑦ ⑧ ⑨ ⑩	☐ Yes...
Mental clarity	① ② ③ ④ ⑤ ⑥ ⑦ ⑧ ⑨ ⑩	

☐ Nausea   ☐ Diarrhea   ☐ Vomiting   ☐ Sore throat
☐ Congestion   ☐ Coughing   ☐ Chills   ☐ Fever

Other symptoms: _____

LAST NIGHT'S SLEEP

Hours of Sleep: _____   Sleep Quality: ① ② ③ ④ ⑤

WEATHER

☐ Hot   ☐ Mild   ☐ Cold   BM Pressure: _____

☐ Dry   ☐ Humid   ☐ Wet   Allergen Levels: _____

☐ Sunny   ☐ Cloudy

STRESS LEVELS

None	Low	Medium	High	Max	@$#%!

FOOD / DRINKS + NON-RELIEF MEDICATION / SUPPLEMENTS

item / meal	time	meds / supplements	dose	time

How many drinks?

water	⟹	① ② ③ ④ ⑤ ⑥ ⑦ ⑧ ⑨ ⑩
caffeine	⟹	① ② ③ ④ ⑤ ⑥ ⑦ ⑧ ⑨ ⑩
alcohol	⟹	① ② ③ ④ ⑤ ⑥ ⑦ ⑧ ⑨ ⑩

HORMONES

☐ Menstruating   ☐ Menopause   ☐ PMS   ☐ N/A | other

COMPUTER USE / READING

☐ None   ☐ Some   ☐ A lot   Total time: [____]

☐ Sitting   ☐ Standing   ☐ Mixture   Breaks every: [____]

PHYSICAL ACTIVITY

☐ None   ☐ Minimal   ☐ Some   ☐ Sweatin'   ☐ I'm beat

DETAILS: _____

RELIEF MEASURES

☐ Medication   ☐ Massage   ☐ Sleep   ☐ Exercise

☐ Water   ☐ Cold/Ice   ☐ Heat/Bath   ☐ Other

DETAILS: _____

DID IT WORK?   ☐ Nope   ☐ A bit   ☐ Mostly   ☐ 100%

Notes

Date:_____

START:	END:	DURATION:

MIGRAINE	CLUSTER	SINUS	TMJ	TENSION

PAIN LEVEL

1	2	3	4	5	6	7	8	9	10

Not too bad.　　　*Well, I'm not enjoying this.*　　　*Holy shit, make it stop!*

DETAILED DESCRIPTION

☐ Constant　　☐ Squeezing　　☐ Throbbing　　☐ Pounding
☐ Dull aching　☐ Burning　　　☐ Sharp　　　☐ Debilitating

Other:_____

ONSET

☐ Slow　　　☐ Average　　☐ Rapid　　☐ Sudden

WHERE DOES IT HURT, EXACTLY?

OTHER SYMPTOMS

☐ Lightheaded　　　☐ Dizziness　　　　☐ Confusion
☐ Light sensitivity　☐ Sound sensitivity　☐ Auras
☐ Muscle stiffness　☐ Muscle burning　　☐ Muscle aches

HOW ARE YOU FEELING OVERALL?　　　　Feeling sick?

Mood	① ② ③ ④ ⑤ ⑥ ⑦ ⑧ ⑨ ⑩	☐ Nope!
Energy levels	① ② ③ ④ ⑤ ⑥ ⑦ ⑧ ⑨ ⑩	☐ Yes...
Mental clarity	① ② ③ ④ ⑤ ⑥ ⑦ ⑧ ⑨ ⑩	

☐ Nausea　　☐ Diarrhea　　☐ Vomiting　　☐ Sore throat
☐ Congestion　☐ Coughing　　☐ Chills　　　☐ Fever

Other symptoms: _____

LAST NIGHT'S SLEEP

Hours of Sleep: _____   Sleep Quality: ① ② ③ ④ ⑤

WEATHER

☐ Hot   ☐ Mild   ☐ Cold   BM Pressure: _____

☐ Dry   ☐ Humid   ☐ Wet   Allergen Levels: _____

☐ Sunny   ☐ Cloudy

STRESS LEVELS

None	Low	Medium	High	Max	@$#%!

FOOD / DRINKS + NON-RELIEF MEDICATION / SUPPLEMENTS

item / meal	time	meds / supplements	dose	time

How many drinks?

water   ① ② ③ ④ ⑤ ⑥ ⑦ ⑧ ⑨ ⑩

caffeine ① ② ③ ④ ⑤ ⑥ ⑦ ⑧ ⑨ ⑩

alcohol ① ② ③ ④ ⑤ ⑥ ⑦ ⑧ ⑨ ⑩

HORMONES

☐ Menstruating   ☐ Menopause   ☐ PMS   ☐ N/A | other

COMPUTER USE / READING

☐ None   ☐ Some   ☐ A lot   Total time: [   ]

☐ Sitting   ☐ Standing   ☐ Mixture   Breaks every: [   ]

PHYSICAL ACTIVITY

☐ None   ☐ Minimal   ☐ Some   ☐ Sweatin'   ☐ I'm beat

DETAILS: _____

RELIEF MEASURES

☐ Medication   ☐ Massage   ☐ Sleep   ☐ Exercise

☐ Water   ☐ Cold/Ice   ☐ Heat/Bath   ☐ Other

DETAILS: _____

DID IT WORK?   ☐ Nope   ☐ A bit   ☐ Mostly   ☐ 100%

Notes

Date:_____

START:	END:	DURATION:

MIGRAINE	CLUSTER	SINUS	TMJ	TENSION

PAIN LEVEL

1	2	3	4	5	6	7	8	9	10

Not too bad.   *Well, I'm not enjoying this.*   *Holy shit, make it stop!*

DETAILED DESCRIPTION

☐ Constant ☐ Squeezing ☐ Throbbing ☐ Pounding
☐ Dull aching ☐ Burning ☐ Sharp ☐ Debilitating

Other:_____

ONSET

☐ Slow ☐ Average ☐ Rapid ☐ Sudden

WHERE DOES IT HURT, EXACTLY?

OTHER SYMPTOMS

☐ Lightheaded ☐ Dizziness ☐ Confusion
☐ Light sensitivity ☐ Sound sensitivity ☐ Auras
☐ Muscle stiffness ☐ Muscle burning ☐ Muscle aches

HOW ARE YOU FEELING OVERALL?

Feeling sick?

Mood ① ② ③ ④ ⑤ ⑥ ⑦ ⑧ ⑨ ⑩	☐ Nope!
Energy levels ① ② ③ ④ ⑤ ⑥ ⑦ ⑧ ⑨ ⑩	☐ Yes...
Mental clarity ① ② ③ ④ ⑤ ⑥ ⑦ ⑧ ⑨ ⑩	

☐ Nausea ☐ Diarrhea ☐ Vomiting ☐ Sore throat
☐ Congestion ☐ Coughing ☐ Chills ☐ Fever

Other symptoms: _____

LAST NIGHT'S SLEEP

Hours of Sleep: _____   Sleep Quality: ① ② ③ ④ ⑤

WEATHER

☐ Hot   ☐ Mild   ☐ Cold   BM Pressure: _____
☐ Dry   ☐ Humid   ☐ Wet   Allergen Levels: _____
☐ Sunny   ☐ Cloudy

STRESS LEVELS

None	Low	Medium	High	Max	@$#%!

FOOD / DRINKS + NON-RELIEF MEDICATION / SUPPLEMENTS

item / meal	time	meds / supplements	dose	time

How many drinks?

water   ① ② ③ ④ ⑤ ⑥ ⑦ ⑧ ⑨ ⑩
caffeine ① ② ③ ④ ⑤ ⑥ ⑦ ⑧ ⑨ ⑩
alcohol   ① ② ③ ④ ⑤ ⑥ ⑦ ⑧ ⑨ ⑩

HORMONES

☐ Menstruating   ☐ Menopause   ☐ PMS   ☐ N/A | other

COMPUTER USE / READING

☐ None   ☐ Some   ☐ A lot   Total time: [   ]
☐ Sitting   ☐ Standing   ☐ Mixture   Breaks every: [   ]

PHYSICAL ACTIVITY

☐ None   ☐ Minimal   ☐ Some   ☐ Sweatin'   ☐ I'm beat
DETAILS: _____

RELIEF MEASURES

☐ Medication   ☐ Massage   ☐ Sleep   ☐ Exercise
☐ Water   ☐ Cold/Ice   ☐ Heat/Bath   ☐ Other
DETAILS: _____

DID IT WORK?   ☐ Nope   ☐ A bit   ☐ Mostly   ☐ 100%

Notes

Date:_____

START:	END:	DURATION:

| MIGRAINE | CLUSTER | SINUS | TMJ | TENSION |

PAIN LEVEL

1	2	3	4	5	6	7	8	9	10

Not too bad.   *Well, I'm not enjoying this.*   *Holy shit, make it stop!*

DETAILED DESCRIPTION

☐ Constant ☐ Squeezing ☐ Throbbing ☐ Pounding
☐ Dull aching ☐ Burning ☐ Sharp ☐ Debilitating

Other:_____

ONSET

☐ Slow ☐ Average ☐ Rapid ☐ Sudden

WHERE DOES IT HURT, EXACTLY?

OTHER SYMPTOMS

☐ Lightheaded ☐ Dizziness ☐ Confusion
☐ Light sensitivity ☐ Sound sensitivity ☐ Auras
☐ Muscle stiffness ☐ Muscle burning ☐ Muscle aches

HOW ARE YOU FEELING OVERALL?

Feeling sick?

Mood	① ② ③ ④ ⑤ ⑥ ⑦ ⑧ ⑨ ⑩	☐ Nope!
Energy levels	① ② ③ ④ ⑤ ⑥ ⑦ ⑧ ⑨ ⑩	☐ Yes...
Mental clarity	① ② ③ ④ ⑤ ⑥ ⑦ ⑧ ⑨ ⑩	

☐ Nausea ☐ Diarrhea ☐ Vomiting ☐ Sore throat
☐ Congestion ☐ Coughing ☐ Chills ☐ Fever

Other symptoms: _____

LAST NIGHT'S SLEEP

Hours of Sleep: _____   Sleep Quality: ① ② ③ ④ ⑤

WEATHER

☐ Hot   ☐ Mild   ☐ Cold   BM Pressure: _____
☐ Dry   ☐ Humid   ☐ Wet   Allergen Levels: _____
☐ Sunny   ☐ Cloudy

STRESS LEVELS

| None | Low | Medium | High | Max | @$#%! |

FOOD / DRINKS + NON-RELIEF MEDICATION / SUPPLEMENTS

item / meal	time	meds / supplements	dose	time

How many drinks?

water   ① ② ③ ④ ⑤ ⑥ ⑦ ⑧ ⑨ ⑩
caffeine ① ② ③ ④ ⑤ ⑥ ⑦ ⑧ ⑨ ⑩
alcohol ① ② ③ ④ ⑤ ⑥ ⑦ ⑧ ⑨ ⑩

HORMONES

☐ Menstruating   ☐ Menopause   ☐ PMS   ☐ N/A | other

COMPUTER USE / READING

☐ None   ☐ Some   ☐ A lot   Total time: [   ]
☐ Sitting   ☐ Standing   ☐ Mixture   Breaks every: [   ]

PHYSICAL ACTIVITY

☐ None   ☐ Minimal   ☐ Some   ☐ Sweatin'   ☐ I'm beat
DETAILS: _____

RELIEF MEASURES

☐ Medication   ☐ Massage   ☐ Sleep   ☐ Exercise
☐ Water   ☐ Cold/Ice   ☐ Heat/Bath   ☐ Other
DETAILS: _____

DID IT WORK?   ☐ Nope   ☐ A bit   ☐ Mostly   ☐ 100%

Notes

Date:_____

START:	END:	DURATION:

MIGRAINE	CLUSTER	SINUS	TMJ	TENSION

PAIN LEVEL

1	2	3	4	5	6	7	8	9	10

Not too bad. *Well, I'm not enjoying this.* *Holy shit, make it stop!*

DETAILED DESCRIPTION

☐ Constant ☐ Squeezing ☐ Throbbing ☐ Pounding
☐ Dull aching ☐ Burning ☐ Sharp ☐ Debilitating

Other:_____

ONSET

☐ Slow ☐ Average ☐ Rapid ☐ Sudden

WHERE DOES IT HURT, EXACTLY?

OTHER SYMPTOMS

☐ Lightheaded ☐ Dizziness ☐ Confusion
☐ Light sensitivity ☐ Sound sensitivity ☐ Auras
☐ Muscle stiffness ☐ Muscle burning ☐ Muscle aches

HOW ARE YOU FEELING OVERALL?

Feeling sick?

Mood	① ② ③ ④ ⑤ ⑥ ⑦ ⑧ ⑨ ⑩	☐ Nope!
Energy levels	① ② ③ ④ ⑤ ⑥ ⑦ ⑧ ⑨ ⑩	☐ Yes...
Mental clarity	① ② ③ ④ ⑤ ⑥ ⑦ ⑧ ⑨ ⑩	

☐ Nausea ☐ Diarrhea ☐ Vomiting ☐ Sore throat
☐ Congestion ☐ Coughing ☐ Chills ☐ Fever

Other symptoms: _____

LAST NIGHT'S SLEEP

Hours of Sleep: _____   Sleep Quality: ① ② ③ ④ ⑤

WEATHER

☐ Hot   ☐ Mild   ☐ Cold   BM Pressure: _____

☐ Dry   ☐ Humid   ☐ Wet   Allergen Levels: _____

☐ Sunny   ☐ Cloudy

STRESS LEVELS

| None | Low | Medium | High | Max | @$#%! |

FOOD / DRINKS + NON-RELIEF MEDICATION / SUPPLEMENTS

item / meal	time	meds / supplements	dose	time

How many drinks?

water → ① ② ③ ④ ⑤ ⑥ ⑦ ⑧ ⑨ ⑩

caffeine → ① ② ③ ④ ⑤ ⑥ ⑦ ⑧ ⑨ ⑩

alcohol → ① ② ③ ④ ⑤ ⑥ ⑦ ⑧ ⑨ ⑩

HORMONES

☐ Menstruating   ☐ Menopause   ☐ PMS   ☐ N/A | other

COMPUTER USE / READING

☐ None   ☐ Some   ☐ A lot   Total time: [   ]

☐ Sitting   ☐ Standing ☐ Mixture   Breaks every: [   ]

PHYSICAL ACTIVITY

☐ None   ☐ Minimal   ☐ Some   ☐ Sweatin'   ☐ I'm beat

DETAILS: _____

RELIEF MEASURES

☐ Medication   ☐ Massage   ☐ Sleep   ☐ Exercise

☐ Water   ☐ Cold/Ice   ☐ Heat/Bath   ☐ Other

DETAILS: _____

DID IT WORK?   ☐ Nope   ☐ A bit   ☐ Mostly   ☐ 100%

Notes

Date:_____

START:	END:	DURATION:

MIGRAINE	CLUSTER	SINUS	TMJ	TENSION

PAIN LEVEL

1	2	3	4	5	6	7	8	9	10

Not too bad.   *Well, I'm not enjoying this.*   *Holy shit, make it stop!*

DETAILED DESCRIPTION

☐ Constant   ☐ Squeezing   ☐ Throbbing   ☐ Pounding
☐ Dull aching   ☐ Burning   ☐ Sharp   ☐ Debilitating

Other:_____

ONSET

☐ Slow   ☐ Average   ☐ Rapid   ☐ Sudden

WHERE DOES IT HURT, EXACTLY?

OTHER SYMPTOMS

☐ Lightheaded   ☐ Dizziness   ☐ Confusion
☐ Light sensitivity ☐ Sound sensitivity ☐ Auras
☐ Muscle stiffness   ☐ Muscle burning   ☐ Muscle aches

HOW ARE YOU FEELING OVERALL?   Feeling sick?

Mood   ① ② ③ ④ ⑤ ⑥ ⑦ ⑧ ⑨ ⑩   ☐ Nope!

Energy levels   ① ② ③ ④ ⑤ ⑥ ⑦ ⑧ ⑨ ⑩   ☐ Yes...

Mental clarity ① ② ③ ④ ⑤ ⑥ ⑦ ⑧ ⑨ ⑩

☐ Nausea   ☐ Diarrhea   ☐ Vomiting   ☐ Sore throat
☐ Congestion   ☐ Coughing   ☐ Chills   ☐ Fever

Other symptoms: _____

LAST NIGHT'S SLEEP
Hours of Sleep: _____   Sleep Quality: ① ② ③ ④ ⑤

WEATHER

☐ Hot   ☐ Mild   ☐ Cold   BM Pressure: _____
☐ Dry   ☐ Humid   ☐ Wet   Allergen Levels: _____
☐ Sunny   ☐ Cloudy

STRESS LEVELS

None	Low	Medium	High	Max	@$#%!

FOOD / DRINKS + NON-RELIEF MEDICATION / SUPPLEMENTS

item / meal	time	meds / supplements	dose	time

How many drinks?

water   ⟹ ① ② ③ ④ ⑤ ⑥ ⑦ ⑧ ⑨ ⑩
caffeine ⟹ ① ② ③ ④ ⑤ ⑥ ⑦ ⑧ ⑨ ⑩
alcohol ⟹ ① ② ③ ④ ⑤ ⑥ ⑦ ⑧ ⑨ ⑩

HORMONES
☐ Menstruating   ☐ Menopause   ☐ PMS   ☐ N/A | other

COMPUTER USE / READING
☐ None   ☐ Some   ☐ A lot   Total time: [   ]
☐ Sitting   ☐ Standing   ☐ Mixture   Breaks every: [   ]

PHYSICAL ACTIVITY
☐ None   ☐ Minimal   ☐ Some   ☐ Sweatin'   ☐ I'm beat
DETAILS: _____

RELIEF MEASURES
☐ Medication   ☐ Massage   ☐ Sleep   ☐ Exercise
☐ Water   ☐ Cold/Ice   ☐ Heat/Bath   ☐ Other
DETAILS: _____

DID IT WORK?   ☐ Nope   ☐ A bit   ☐ Mostly   ☐ 100%

Notes

Date:_____

START:	END:	DURATION:

| MIGRAINE | CLUSTER | SINUS | TMJ | TENSION |

PAIN LEVEL

1	2	3	4	5	6	7	8	9	10

Not too bad.   *Well, I'm not enjoying this.*   *Holy shit, make it stop!*

DETAILED DESCRIPTION

☐ Constant   ☐ Squeezing   ☐ Throbbing   ☐ Pounding
☐ Dull aching ☐ Burning   ☐ Sharp   ☐ Debilitating

Other:_____

ONSET

☐ Slow   ☐ Average   ☐ Rapid   ☐ Sudden

WHERE DOES IT HURT, EXACTLY?

OTHER SYMPTOMS

☐ Lightheaded   ☐ Dizziness   ☐ Confusion
☐ Light sensitivity ☐ Sound sensitivity ☐ Auras
☐ Muscle stiffness ☐ Muscle burning   ☐ Muscle aches

HOW ARE YOU FEELING OVERALL?   Feeling sick?

Mood	① ② ③ ④ ⑤ ⑥ ⑦ ⑧ ⑨ ⑩	☐ Nope!
Energy levels	① ② ③ ④ ⑤ ⑥ ⑦ ⑧ ⑨ ⑩	☐ Yes...
Mental clarity	① ② ③ ④ ⑤ ⑥ ⑦ ⑧ ⑨ ⑩	

☐ Nausea   ☐ Diarrhea   ☐ Vomiting   ☐ Sore throat
☐ Congestion ☐ Coughing   ☐ Chills   ☐ Fever

Other symptoms: _____

LAST NIGHT'S SLEEP

Hours of Sleep: _____   Sleep Quality: ① ② ③ ④ ⑤

WEATHER

☐ Hot   ☐ Mild   ☐ Cold   BM Pressure: _____

☐ Dry   ☐ Humid   ☐ Wet   Allergen Levels: _____

☐ Sunny   ☐ Cloudy

STRESS LEVELS

None	Low	Medium	High	Max	@$#%!

FOOD / DRINKS + NON-RELIEF MEDICATION / SUPPLEMENTS

item / meal	time	meds / supplements	dose	time

How many drinks?

water	① ② ③ ④ ⑤ ⑥ ⑦ ⑧ ⑨ ⑩
caffeine	① ② ③ ④ ⑤ ⑥ ⑦ ⑧ ⑨ ⑩
alcohol	① ② ③ ④ ⑤ ⑥ ⑦ ⑧ ⑨ ⑩

HORMONES

☐ Menstruating   ☐ Menopause   ☐ PMS   ☐ N/A | other

COMPUTER USE / READING

☐ None   ☐ Some   ☐ A lot   Total time: [   ]

☐ Sitting   ☐ Standing   ☐ Mixture   Breaks every: [   ]

PHYSICAL ACTIVITY

☐ None   ☐ Minimal   ☐ Some   ☐ Sweatin'   ☐ I'm beat

DETAILS: _____

RELIEF MEASURES

☐ Medication   ☐ Massage   ☐ Sleep   ☐ Exercise

☐ Water   ☐ Cold/Ice   ☐ Heat/Bath   ☐ Other

DETAILS: _____

DID IT WORK?   ☐ Nope   ☐ A bit   ☐ Mostly   ☐ 100%

Notes

Date:_____

START:	END:	DURATION:

MIGRAINE CLUSTER SINUS TMJ TENSION

PAIN LEVEL

1	2	3	4	5	6	7	8	9	10

Not too bad.   *Well, I'm not enjoying this.*   *Holy shit, make it stop!*

DETAILED DESCRIPTION

☐ Constant ☐ Squeezing ☐ Throbbing ☐ Pounding
☐ Dull aching ☐ Burning ☐ Sharp ☐ Debilitating

Other:_____

ONSET

☐ Slow ☐ Average ☐ Rapid ☐ Sudden

WHERE DOES IT HURT, EXACTLY?

OTHER SYMPTOMS

☐ Lightheaded ☐ Dizziness ☐ Confusion
☐ Light sensitivity ☐ Sound sensitivity ☐ Auras
☐ Muscle stiffness ☐ Muscle burning ☐ Muscle aches

HOW ARE YOU FEELING OVERALL?

Feeling sick?

Mood   ① ② ③ ④ ⑤ ⑥ ⑦ ⑧ ⑨ ⑩   ☐ Nope!
Energy levels   ① ② ③ ④ ⑤ ⑥ ⑦ ⑧ ⑨ ⑩   ☐ Yes...
Mental clarity ① ② ③ ④ ⑤ ⑥ ⑦ ⑧ ⑨ ⑩

☐ Nausea ☐ Diarrhea ☐ Vomiting ☐ Sore throat
☐ Congestion ☐ Coughing ☐ Chills ☐ Fever

Other symptoms: _____

LAST NIGHT'S SLEEP

Hours of Sleep: _____   Sleep Quality: ① ② ③ ④ ⑤

WEATHER

☐ Hot   ☐ Mild   ☐ Cold   BM Pressure: _____

☐ Dry   ☐ Humid   ☐ Wet   Allergen Levels: _____

☐ Sunny   ☐ Cloudy

STRESS LEVELS

None	Low	Medium	High	Max	@$#%!

FOOD / DRINKS + NON-RELIEF MEDICATION / SUPPLEMENTS

item / meal	time	meds / supplements	dose	time

How many drinks?

water   ① ② ③ ④ ⑤ ⑥ ⑦ ⑧ ⑨ ⑩

caffeine ① ② ③ ④ ⑤ ⑥ ⑦ ⑧ ⑨ ⑩

alcohol ① ② ③ ④ ⑤ ⑥ ⑦ ⑧ ⑨ ⑩

HORMONES

☐ Menstruating   ☐ Menopause   ☐ PMS   ☐ N/A | other

COMPUTER USE / READING

☐ None   ☐ Some   ☐ A lot   Total time: [   ]

☐ Sitting   ☐ Standing   ☐ Mixture   Breaks every: [   ]

PHYSICAL ACTIVITY

☐ None   ☐ Minimal   ☐ Some   ☐ Sweatin'   ☐ I'm beat

DETAILS: _____

RELIEF MEASURES

☐ Medication   ☐ Massage   ☐ Sleep   ☐ Exercise

☐ Water   ☐ Cold/Ice   ☐ Heat/Bath   ☐ Other

DETAILS: _____

DID IT WORK?   ☐ Nope   ☐ A bit   ☐ Mostly   ☐ 100%

Notes

Date:_____

START:	END:	DURATION:

MIGRAINE	CLUSTER	SINUS	TMJ	TENSION

PAIN LEVEL

1	2	3	4	5	6	7	8	9	10

Not too bad.　　　*Well, I'm not enjoying this.*　　　*Holy shit, make it stop!*

DETAILED DESCRIPTION

☐ Constant　　☐ Squeezing　　☐ Throbbing　　☐ Pounding
☐ Dull aching　☐ Burning　　　☐ Sharp　　　　☐ Debilitating

Other:_____

ONSET

☐ Slow　　　☐ Average　　☐ Rapid　　☐ Sudden

WHERE DOES IT HURT, EXACTLY?

OTHER SYMPTOMS

☐ Lightheaded　　　☐ Dizziness　　　　☐ Confusion
☐ Light sensitivity　☐ Sound sensitivity　☐ Auras
☐ Muscle stiffness　☐ Muscle burning　　☐ Muscle aches

HOW ARE YOU FEELING OVERALL?　　　Feeling sick?

Mood ① ② ③ ④ ⑤ ⑥ ⑦ ⑧ ⑨ ⑩　　☐ Nope!

Energy levels ① ② ③ ④ ⑤ ⑥ ⑦ ⑧ ⑨ ⑩　☐ Yes...

Mental clarity ① ② ③ ④ ⑤ ⑥ ⑦ ⑧ ⑨ ⑩

☐ Nausea　　　☐ Diarrhea　☐ Vomiting　☐ Sore throat
☐ Congestion　☐ Coughing　☐ Chills　　☐ Fever

Other symptoms: _____

LAST NIGHT'S SLEEP

Hours of Sleep: _____   Sleep Quality: ① ② ③ ④ ⑤

WEATHER

☐ Hot   ☐ Mild   ☐ Cold   BM Pressure: _____

☐ Dry   ☐ Humid   ☐ Wet   Allergen Levels: _____

☐ Sunny   ☐ Cloudy

STRESS LEVELS

None	Low	Medium	High	Max	@$#%!

FOOD / DRINKS + NON-RELIEF MEDICATION / SUPPLEMENTS

item / meal	time	meds / supplements	dose	time

How many drinks?

water   ① ② ③ ④ ⑤ ⑥ ⑦ ⑧ ⑨ ⑩

caffeine ① ② ③ ④ ⑤ ⑥ ⑦ ⑧ ⑨ ⑩

alcohol ① ② ③ ④ ⑤ ⑥ ⑦ ⑧ ⑨ ⑩

HORMONES

☐ Menstruating   ☐ Menopause   ☐ PMS   ☐ N/A | other

COMPUTER USE / READING

☐ None   ☐ Some   ☐ A lot   Total time: [   ]

☐ Sitting   ☐ Standing   ☐ Mixture   Breaks every: [   ]

PHYSICAL ACTIVITY

☐ None   ☐ Minimal   ☐ Some   ☐ Sweatin'   ☐ I'm beat

DETAILS: _____

RELIEF MEASURES

☐ Medication   ☐ Massage   ☐ Sleep   ☐ Exercise

☐ Water   ☐ Cold/Ice   ☐ Heat/Bath   ☐ Other

DETAILS: _____

DID IT WORK?   ☐ Nope   ☐ A bit   ☐ Mostly   ☐ 100%

Notes

Date:_____

| START: | END: | DURATION: |

| MIGRAINE | CLUSTER | SINUS | TMJ | TENSION |

PAIN LEVEL

| 1 | 2 | 3 | 4 | 5 | 6 | 7 | 8 | 9 | 10 |

Not too bad.   *Well, I'm not enjoying this.*   *Holy shit, make it stop!*

DETAILED DESCRIPTION

☐ Constant ☐ Squeezing ☐ Throbbing ☐ Pounding
☐ Dull aching ☐ Burning ☐ Sharp ☐ Debilitating

Other:_____

ONSET

☐ Slow ☐ Average ☐ Rapid ☐ Sudden

WHERE DOES IT HURT, EXACTLY?

OTHER SYMPTOMS

☐ Lightheaded ☐ Dizziness ☐ Confusion
☐ Light sensitivity ☐ Sound sensitivity ☐ Auras
☐ Muscle stiffness ☐ Muscle burning ☐ Muscle aches

HOW ARE YOU FEELING OVERALL?   Feeling sick?

Mood   ① ② ③ ④ ⑤ ⑥ ⑦ ⑧ ⑨ ⑩   ☐ Nope!

Energy levels   ① ② ③ ④ ⑤ ⑥ ⑦ ⑧ ⑨ ⑩   ☐ Yes...

Mental clarity   ① ② ③ ④ ⑤ ⑥ ⑦ ⑧ ⑨ ⑩

☐ Nausea ☐ Diarrhea ☐ Vomiting ☐ Sore throat
☐ Congestion ☐ Coughing ☐ Chills ☐ Fever

Other symptoms: _____

LAST NIGHT'S SLEEP

Hours of Sleep: _____   Sleep Quality: ① ② ③ ④ ⑤

WEATHER

☐ Hot   ☐ Mild   ☐ Cold   BM Pressure: _____

☐ Dry   ☐ Humid   ☐ Wet   Allergen Levels: _____

☐ Sunny   ☐ Cloudy

STRESS LEVELS

None	Low	Medium	High	Max	@$#%!

FOOD / DRINKS + NON-RELIEF MEDICATION / SUPPLEMENTS

item / meal	time	meds / supplements	dose	time

How many drinks?

water   ① ② ③ ④ ⑤ ⑥ ⑦ ⑧ ⑨ ⑩

caffeine   ① ② ③ ④ ⑤ ⑥ ⑦ ⑧ ⑨ ⑩

alcohol   ① ② ③ ④ ⑤ ⑥ ⑦ ⑧ ⑨ ⑩

HORMONES

☐ Menstruating   ☐ Menopause   ☐ PMS   ☐ N/A | other

COMPUTER USE / READING

☐ None   ☐ Some   ☐ A lot   Total time: [＿＿]

☐ Sitting   ☐ Standing   ☐ Mixture   Breaks every: [＿＿]

PHYSICAL ACTIVITY

☐ None   ☐ Minimal   ☐ Some   ☐ Sweatin'   ☐ I'm beat

DETAILS: _____

RELIEF MEASURES

☐ Medication   ☐ Massage   ☐ Sleep   ☐ Exercise

☐ Water   ☐ Cold/Ice   ☐ Heat/Bath   ☐ Other

DETAILS: _____

DID IT WORK?   ☐ Nope   ☐ A bit   ☐ Mostly   ☐ 100%

Notes

Date:_____

START:	END:	DURATION:

MIGRAINE	CLUSTER	SINUS	TMJ	TENSION

PAIN LEVEL

1	2	3	4	5	6	7	8	9	10

Not too bad. *Well, I'm not enjoying this.* *Holy shit, make it stop!*

DETAILED DESCRIPTION

☐ Constant ☐ Squeezing ☐ Throbbing ☐ Pounding
☐ Dull aching ☐ Burning ☐ Sharp ☐ Debilitating

Other:_____

ONSET

☐ Slow ☐ Average ☐ Rapid ☐ Sudden

WHERE DOES IT HURT, EXACTLY?

OTHER SYMPTOMS

☐ Lightheaded ☐ Dizziness ☐ Confusion
☐ Light sensitivity ☐ Sound sensitivity ☐ Auras
☐ Muscle stiffness ☐ Muscle burning ☐ Muscle aches

HOW ARE YOU FEELING OVERALL? Feeling sick?

Mood ① ② ③ ④ ⑤ ⑥ ⑦ ⑧ ⑨ ⑩ ☐ Nope!

Energy levels ① ② ③ ④ ⑤ ⑥ ⑦ ⑧ ⑨ ⑩ ☐ Yes...

Mental clarity ① ② ③ ④ ⑤ ⑥ ⑦ ⑧ ⑨ ⑩

☐ Nausea ☐ Diarrhea ☐ Vomiting ☐ Sore throat
☐ Congestion ☐ Coughing ☐ Chills ☐ Fever

Other symptoms: _____

LAST NIGHT'S SLEEP

Hours of Sleep: _____   Sleep Quality: ① ② ③ ④ ⑤

WEATHER

☐ Hot   ☐ Mild   ☐ Cold   BM Pressure: _____

☐ Dry   ☐ Humid   ☐ Wet   Allergen Levels: _____

☐ Sunny   ☐ Cloudy

STRESS LEVELS

None	Low	Medium	High	Max	@$#%!

FOOD / DRINKS + NON-RELIEF MEDICATION / SUPPLEMENTS

item / meal	time	meds / supplements	dose	time

How many drinks?

water		① ② ③ ④ ⑤ ⑥ ⑦ ⑧ ⑨ ⑩
caffeine		① ② ③ ④ ⑤ ⑥ ⑦ ⑧ ⑨ ⑩
alcohol		① ② ③ ④ ⑤ ⑥ ⑦ ⑧ ⑨ ⑩

HORMONES

☐ Menstruating   ☐ Menopause   ☐ PMS   ☐ N/A | other

COMPUTER USE / READING

☐ None   ☐ Some   ☐ A lot   Total time: [   ]

☐ Sitting   ☐ Standing   ☐ Mixture   Breaks every: [   ]

PHYSICAL ACTIVITY

☐ None   ☐ Minimal   ☐ Some   ☐ Sweatin'   ☐ I'm beat

DETAILS: _____

RELIEF MEASURES

☐ Medication   ☐ Massage   ☐ Sleep   ☐ Exercise

☐ Water   ☐ Cold/Ice   ☐ Heat/Bath   ☐ Other

DETAILS: _____

DID IT WORK?   ☐ Nope   ☐ A bit   ☐ Mostly   ☐ 100%

Notes

Date:_____

START:	END:	DURATION:

MIGRAINE	CLUSTER	SINUS	TMJ	TENSION

PAIN LEVEL

1	2	3	4	5	6	7	8	9	10

Not too bad.   *Well, I'm not enjoying this.*   *Holy shit, make it stop!*

DETAILED DESCRIPTION

☐ Constant   ☐ Squeezing   ☐ Throbbing   ☐ Pounding
☐ Dull aching   ☐ Burning   ☐ Sharp   ☐ Debilitating

Other:_____

ONSET

☐ Slow   ☐ Average   ☐ Rapid   ☐ Sudden

WHERE DOES IT HURT, EXACTLY?

OTHER SYMPTOMS

☐ Lightheaded   ☐ Dizziness   ☐ Confusion
☐ Light sensitivity   ☐ Sound sensitivity   ☐ Auras
☐ Muscle stiffness   ☐ Muscle burning   ☐ Muscle aches

HOW ARE YOU FEELING OVERALL?

Feeling sick?

Mood	① ② ③ ④ ⑤ ⑥ ⑦ ⑧ ⑨ ⑩	☐ Nope!
Energy levels	① ② ③ ④ ⑤ ⑥ ⑦ ⑧ ⑨ ⑩	☐ Yes...
Mental clarity	① ② ③ ④ ⑤ ⑥ ⑦ ⑧ ⑨ ⑩	

☐ Nausea   ☐ Diarrhea   ☐ Vomiting   ☐ Sore throat
☐ Congestion   ☐ Coughing   ☐ Chills   ☐ Fever

Other symptoms: _____

LAST NIGHT'S SLEEP

Hours of Sleep: _____   Sleep Quality: ① ② ③ ④ ⑤

WEATHER

☐ Hot   ☐ Mild   ☐ Cold   BM Pressure: _____

☐ Dry   ☐ Humid   ☐ Wet   Allergen Levels: _____

☐ Sunny   ☐ Cloudy

STRESS LEVELS

None	Low	Medium	High	Max	@$#%!

FOOD / DRINKS + NON-RELIEF MEDICATION / SUPPLEMENTS

item / meal	time	meds / supplements	dose	time

How many drinks?

water	① ② ③ ④ ⑤ ⑥ ⑦ ⑧ ⑨ ⑩
caffeine	① ② ③ ④ ⑤ ⑥ ⑦ ⑧ ⑨ ⑩
alcohol	① ② ③ ④ ⑤ ⑥ ⑦ ⑧ ⑨ ⑩

HORMONES

☐ Menstruating   ☐ Menopause   ☐ PMS   ☐ N/A | other

COMPUTER USE / READING

☐ None   ☐ Some   ☐ A lot   Total time: [   ]

☐ Sitting   ☐ Standing   ☐ Mixture   Breaks every: [   ]

PHYSICAL ACTIVITY

☐ None   ☐ Minimal   ☐ Some   ☐ Sweatin'   ☐ I'm beat

DETAILS: _____

RELIEF MEASURES

☐ Medication   ☐ Massage   ☐ Sleep   ☐ Exercise

☐ Water   ☐ Cold/Ice   ☐ Heat/Bath   ☐ Other

DETAILS: _____

DID IT WORK?   ☐ Nope   ☐ A bit   ☐ Mostly   ☐ 100%

Notes

Date:_____

| START: | END: | DURATION: |

| MIGRAINE | CLUSTER | SINUS | TMJ | TENSION |

PAIN LEVEL

1	2	3	4	5	6	7	8	9	10

Not too bad. *Well, I'm not enjoying this.* *Holy shit, make it stop!*

DETAILED DESCRIPTION

☐ Constant ☐ Squeezing ☐ Throbbing ☐ Pounding
☐ Dull aching ☐ Burning ☐ Sharp ☐ Debilitating

Other:_____

ONSET

☐ Slow ☐ Average ☐ Rapid ☐ Sudden

WHERE DOES IT HURT, EXACTLY?

OTHER SYMPTOMS

☐ Lightheaded ☐ Dizziness ☐ Confusion
☐ Light sensitivity ☐ Sound sensitivity ☐ Auras
☐ Muscle stiffness ☐ Muscle burning ☐ Muscle aches

HOW ARE YOU FEELING OVERALL?

Feeling sick?

Mood ①②③④⑤⑥⑦⑧⑨⑩ ☐ Nope!

Energy levels ①②③④⑤⑥⑦⑧⑨⑩ ☐ Yes...

Mental clarity ①②③④⑤⑥⑦⑧⑨⑩

☐ Nausea ☐ Diarrhea ☐ Vomiting ☐ Sore throat
☐ Congestion ☐ Coughing ☐ Chills ☐ Fever

Other symptoms: _____

LAST NIGHT'S SLEEP

Hours of Sleep: _____   Sleep Quality: ① ② ③ ④ ⑤

WEATHER

☐ Hot   ☐ Mild   ☐ Cold   BM Pressure: _____

☐ Dry   ☐ Humid   ☐ Wet   Allergen Levels: _____

☐ Sunny   ☐ Cloudy

STRESS LEVELS

None	Low	Medium	High	Max	@$#%!

FOOD / DRINKS + NON-RELIEF MEDICATION / SUPPLEMENTS

item / meal	time	meds / supplements	dose	time

How many drinks?

water   ① ② ③ ④ ⑤ ⑥ ⑦ ⑧ ⑨ ⑩

caffeine ① ② ③ ④ ⑤ ⑥ ⑦ ⑧ ⑨ ⑩

alcohol   ① ② ③ ④ ⑤ ⑥ ⑦ ⑧ ⑨ ⑩

HORMONES

☐ Menstruating   ☐ Menopause   ☐ PMS   ☐ N/A | other

COMPUTER USE / READING

☐ None   ☐ Some   ☐ A lot   Total time: [   ]

☐ Sitting   ☐ Standing   ☐ Mixture   Breaks every: [   ]

PHYSICAL ACTIVITY

☐ None   ☐ Minimal   ☐ Some   ☐ Sweatin'   ☐ I'm beat

DETAILS: _____

RELIEF MEASURES

☐ Medication ☐ Massage   ☐ Sleep   ☐ Exercise

☐ Water   ☐ Cold/Ice   ☐ Heat/Bath   ☐ Other

DETAILS: _____

DID IT WORK?   ☐ Nope   ☐ A bit   ☐ Mostly   ☐ 100%

Notes

Date:_____

START:	END:	DURATION:

MIGRAINE	CLUSTER	SINUS	TMJ	TENSION

PAIN LEVEL

1	2	3	4	5	6	7	8	9	10

Not too bad.   *Well, I'm not enjoying this.*   *Holy shit, make it stop!*

DETAILED DESCRIPTION

☐ Constant   ☐ Squeezing   ☐ Throbbing   ☐ Pounding
☐ Dull aching   ☐ Burning   ☐ Sharp   ☐ Debilitating

Other:_____

ONSET

☐ Slow   ☐ Average   ☐ Rapid   ☐ Sudden

WHERE DOES IT HURT, EXACTLY?

OTHER SYMPTOMS

☐ Lightheaded   ☐ Dizziness   ☐ Confusion
☐ Light sensitivity   ☐ Sound sensitivity   ☐ Auras
☐ Muscle stiffness   ☐ Muscle burning   ☐ Muscle aches

HOW ARE YOU FEELING OVERALL?

Feeling sick?

Mood ① ② ③ ④ ⑤ ⑥ ⑦ ⑧ ⑨ ⑩   ☐ Nope!

Energy levels ① ② ③ ④ ⑤ ⑥ ⑦ ⑧ ⑨ ⑩   ☐ Yes...

Mental clarity ① ② ③ ④ ⑤ ⑥ ⑦ ⑧ ⑨ ⑩

☐ Nausea   ☐ Diarrhea   ☐ Vomiting   ☐ Sore throat
☐ Congestion   ☐ Coughing   ☐ Chills   ☐ Fever

Other symptoms: _____

LAST NIGHT'S SLEEP

Hours of Sleep: _____   Sleep Quality: ① ② ③ ④ ⑤

WEATHER

☐ Hot   ☐ Mild   ☐ Cold   BM Pressure: _____
☐ Dry   ☐ Humid   ☐ Wet   Allergen Levels: _____
☐ Sunny   ☐ Cloudy

STRESS LEVELS

None	Low	Medium	High	Max	@$#%!

FOOD / DRINKS + NON-RELIEF MEDICATION / SUPPLEMENTS

item / meal	time	meds / supplements	dose	time

How many drinks?

water   ① ② ③ ④ ⑤ ⑥ ⑦ ⑧ ⑨ ⑩
caffeine ① ② ③ ④ ⑤ ⑥ ⑦ ⑧ ⑨ ⑩
alcohol   ① ② ③ ④ ⑤ ⑥ ⑦ ⑧ ⑨ ⑩

HORMONES

☐ Menstruating   ☐ Menopause   ☐ PMS   ☐ N/A | other

COMPUTER USE / READING

☐ None   ☐ Some   ☐ A lot   Total time: [   ]
☐ Sitting   ☐ Standing   ☐ Mixture   Breaks every: [   ]

PHYSICAL ACTIVITY

☐ None   ☐ Minimal   ☐ Some   ☐ Sweatin'   ☐ I'm beat
DETAILS: _____

RELIEF MEASURES

☐ Medication   ☐ Massage   ☐ Sleep   ☐ Exercise
☐ Water   ☐ Cold/Ice   ☐ Heat/Bath   ☐ Other
DETAILS: _____

DID IT WORK?   ☐ Nope   ☐ A bit   ☐ Mostly   ☐ 100%

Notes

Date:_____

START:	END:	DURATION:

MIGRAINE	CLUSTER	SINUS	TMJ	TENSION

PAIN LEVEL

1	2	3	4	5	6	7	8	9	10

Not too bad.   *Well, I'm not enjoying this.*   *Holy shit, make it stop!*

DETAILED DESCRIPTION

☐ Constant   ☐ Squeezing   ☐ Throbbing   ☐ Pounding
☐ Dull aching   ☐ Burning   ☐ Sharp   ☐ Debilitating

Other:_____

ONSET

☐ Slow   ☐ Average   ☐ Rapid   ☐ Sudden

WHERE DOES IT HURT, EXACTLY?

OTHER SYMPTOMS

☐ Lightheaded   ☐ Dizziness   ☐ Confusion
☐ Light sensitivity ☐ Sound sensitivity   ☐ Auras
☐ Muscle stiffness   ☐ Muscle burning   ☐ Muscle aches

HOW ARE YOU FEELING OVERALL?   Feeling sick?

Mood   ① ② ③ ④ ⑤ ⑥ ⑦ ⑧ ⑨ ⑩   ☐ Nope!

Energy levels   ① ② ③ ④ ⑤ ⑥ ⑦ ⑧ ⑨ ⑩   ☐ Yes...

Mental clarity ① ② ③ ④ ⑤ ⑥ ⑦ ⑧ ⑨ ⑩

☐ Nausea   ☐ Diarrhea   ☐ Vomiting   ☐ Sore throat
☐ Congestion   ☐ Coughing   ☐ Chills   ☐ Fever

Other symptoms: _____

LAST NIGHT'S SLEEP

Hours of Sleep: _____   Sleep Quality: ① ② ③ ④ ⑤

WEATHER

☐ Hot   ☐ Mild   ☐ Cold   BM Pressure: _____

☐ Dry   ☐ Humid   ☐ Wet   Allergen Levels: _____

☐ Sunny   ☐ Cloudy

STRESS LEVELS

None	Low	Medium	High	Max	@$#%!

FOOD / DRINKS + NON-RELIEF MEDICATION / SUPPLEMENTS

item / meal	time	meds / supplements	dose	time

How many drinks?

water	→	① ② ③ ④ ⑤ ⑥ ⑦ ⑧ ⑨ ⑩
caffeine	→	① ② ③ ④ ⑤ ⑥ ⑦ ⑧ ⑨ ⑩
alcohol	→	① ② ③ ④ ⑤ ⑥ ⑦ ⑧ ⑨ ⑩

HORMONES

☐ Menstruating   ☐ Menopause   ☐ PMS   ☐ N/A | other

COMPUTER USE / READING

☐ None   ☐ Some   ☐ A lot   Total time: [____]

☐ Sitting   ☐ Standing   ☐ Mixture   Breaks every: [____]

PHYSICAL ACTIVITY

☐ None   ☐ Minimal   ☐ Some   ☐ Sweatin'   ☐ I'm beat

DETAILS: _____

RELIEF MEASURES

☐ Medication   ☐ Massage   ☐ Sleep   ☐ Exercise

☐ Water   ☐ Cold/Ice   ☐ Heat/Bath   ☐ Other

DETAILS: _____

DID IT WORK?   ☐ Nope   ☐ A bit   ☐ Mostly   ☐ 100%

Notes

Date:_____

START:	END:	DURATION:

| MIGRAINE | CLUSTER | SINUS | TMJ | TENSION |

PAIN LEVEL

1	2	3	4	5	6	7	8	9	10

Not too bad.   *Well, I'm not enjoying this.*   *Holy shit, make it stop!*

DETAILED DESCRIPTION

☐ Constant   ☐ Squeezing   ☐ Throbbing   ☐ Pounding
☐ Dull aching   ☐ Burning   ☐ Sharp   ☐ Debilitating

Other:_____

ONSET

☐ Slow   ☐ Average   ☐ Rapid   ☐ Sudden

WHERE DOES IT HURT, EXACTLY?

OTHER SYMPTOMS

☐ Lightheaded   ☐ Dizziness   ☐ Confusion
☐ Light sensitivity ☐ Sound sensitivity ☐ Auras
☐ Muscle stiffness ☐ Muscle burning   ☐ Muscle aches

HOW ARE YOU FEELING OVERALL?   Feeling sick?

Mood   ① ② ③ ④ ⑤ ⑥ ⑦ ⑧ ⑨ ⑩   ☐ Nope!
Energy levels   ① ② ③ ④ ⑤ ⑥ ⑦ ⑧ ⑨ ⑩   ☐ Yes...
Mental clarity ① ② ③ ④ ⑤ ⑥ ⑦ ⑧ ⑨ ⑩

☐ Nausea   ☐ Diarrhea   ☐ Vomiting   ☐ Sore throat
☐ Congestion   ☐ Coughing   ☐ Chills   ☐ Fever

Other symptoms: _____

LAST NIGHT'S SLEEP

Hours of Sleep: _____   Sleep Quality: ① ② ③ ④ ⑤

WEATHER

☐ Hot   ☐ Mild   ☐ Cold   BM Pressure: _____

☐ Dry   ☐ Humid   ☐ Wet   Allergen Levels: _____

☐ Sunny   ☐ Cloudy

STRESS LEVELS

None	Low	Medium	High	Max	@$#%!

FOOD / DRINKS + NON-RELIEF MEDICATION / SUPPLEMENTS

item / meal	time	meds / supplements	dose	time

How many drinks?

water → ① ② ③ ④ ⑤ ⑥ ⑦ ⑧ ⑨ ⑩

caffeine → ① ② ③ ④ ⑤ ⑥ ⑦ ⑧ ⑨ ⑩

alcohol → ① ② ③ ④ ⑤ ⑥ ⑦ ⑧ ⑨ ⑩

HORMONES

☐ Menstruating   ☐ Menopause   ☐ PMS   ☐ N/A | other

COMPUTER USE / READING

☐ None   ☐ Some   ☐ A lot   Total time: [   ]

☐ Sitting   ☐ Standing   ☐ Mixture   Breaks every: [   ]

PHYSICAL ACTIVITY

☐ None   ☐ Minimal   ☐ Some   ☐ Sweatin'   ☐ I'm beat

DETAILS: _____

RELIEF MEASURES

☐ Medication   ☐ Massage   ☐ Sleep   ☐ Exercise

☐ Water   ☐ Cold/Ice   ☐ Heat/Bath   ☐ Other

DETAILS: _____

DID IT WORK?   ☐ Nope   ☐ A bit   ☐ Mostly   ☐ 100%

Notes

Date:_____

START:	END:	DURATION:

| MIGRAINE | CLUSTER | SINUS | TMJ | TENSION |

PAIN LEVEL

1	2	3	4	5	6	7	8	9	10

Not too bad.   *Well, I'm not enjoying this.*   *Holy shit, make it stop!*

DETAILED DESCRIPTION

☐ Constant   ☐ Squeezing   ☐ Throbbing   ☐ Pounding
☐ Dull aching   ☐ Burning   ☐ Sharp   ☐ Debilitating

Other:_____

ONSET

☐ Slow   ☐ Average   ☐ Rapid   ☐ Sudden

WHERE DOES IT HURT, EXACTLY?

OTHER SYMPTOMS

☐ Lightheaded   ☐ Dizziness   ☐ Confusion
☐ Light sensitivity   ☐ Sound sensitivity   ☐ Auras
☐ Muscle stiffness   ☐ Muscle burning   ☐ Muscle aches

HOW ARE YOU FEELING OVERALL?

Feeling sick?

Mood	① ② ③ ④ ⑤ ⑥ ⑦ ⑧ ⑨ ⑩	☐ Nope!
Energy levels	① ② ③ ④ ⑤ ⑥ ⑦ ⑧ ⑨ ⑩	☐ Yes...
Mental clarity	① ② ③ ④ ⑤ ⑥ ⑦ ⑧ ⑨ ⑩	

☐ Nausea   ☐ Diarrhea   ☐ Vomiting   ☐ Sore throat
☐ Congestion   ☐ Coughing   ☐ Chills   ☐ Fever

Other symptoms: _____

LAST NIGHT'S SLEEP

Hours of Sleep: _____   Sleep Quality: ① ② ③ ④ ⑤

WEATHER

☐ Hot   ☐ Mild   ☐ Cold   BM Pressure: _____

☐ Dry   ☐ Humid   ☐ Wet   Allergen Levels: _____

☐ Sunny   ☐ Cloudy

STRESS LEVELS

None	Low	Medium	High	Max	@$#%!

FOOD / DRINKS + NON-RELIEF MEDICATION / SUPPLEMENTS

item / meal	time	meds / supplements	dose	time

How many drinks?

water   → ① ② ③ ④ ⑤ ⑥ ⑦ ⑧ ⑨ ⑩

caffeine → ① ② ③ ④ ⑤ ⑥ ⑦ ⑧ ⑨ ⑩

alcohol → ① ② ③ ④ ⑤ ⑥ ⑦ ⑧ ⑨ ⑩

HORMONES

☐ Menstruating   ☐ Menopause   ☐ PMS   ☐ N/A | other

COMPUTER USE / READING

☐ None   ☐ Some   ☐ A lot   Total time: [____]

☐ Sitting   ☐ Standing   ☐ Mixture   Breaks every: [____]

PHYSICAL ACTIVITY

☐ None   ☐ Minimal   ☐ Some   ☐ Sweatin'   ☐ I'm beat

DETAILS: _____

RELIEF MEASURES

☐ Medication   ☐ Massage   ☐ Sleep   ☐ Exercise

☐ Water   ☐ Cold/Ice   ☐ Heat/Bath   ☐ Other

DETAILS: _____

DID IT WORK?   ☐ Nope   ☐ A bit   ☐ Mostly   ☐ 100%

Notes

Date:_____

START:	END:	DURATION:

MIGRAINE	CLUSTER	SINUS	TMJ	TENSION

PAIN LEVEL

1	2	3	4	5	6	7	8	9	10

Not too bad.   *Well, I'm not enjoying this.*   *Holy shit, make it stop!*

DETAILED DESCRIPTION

☐ Constant   ☐ Squeezing   ☐ Throbbing   ☐ Pounding
☐ Dull aching   ☐ Burning   ☐ Sharp   ☐ Debilitating

Other:_____

ONSET

☐ Slow   ☐ Average   ☐ Rapid   ☐ Sudden

WHERE DOES IT HURT, EXACTLY?

OTHER SYMPTOMS

☐ Lightheaded   ☐ Dizziness   ☐ Confusion
☐ Light sensitivity   ☐ Sound sensitivity   ☐ Auras
☐ Muscle stiffness   ☐ Muscle burning   ☐ Muscle aches

HOW ARE YOU FEELING OVERALL?   Feeling sick?

Mood	① ② ③ ④ ⑤ ⑥ ⑦ ⑧ ⑨ ⑩	☐ Nope!
Energy levels	① ② ③ ④ ⑤ ⑥ ⑦ ⑧ ⑨ ⑩	☐ Yes...
Mental clarity	① ② ③ ④ ⑤ ⑥ ⑦ ⑧ ⑨ ⑩	

☐ Nausea   ☐ Diarrhea   ☐ Vomiting   ☐ Sore throat
☐ Congestion   ☐ Coughing   ☐ Chills   ☐ Fever

Other symptoms: _____

LAST NIGHT'S SLEEP

Hours of Sleep: _____   Sleep Quality: ① ② ③ ④ ⑤

WEATHER

☐ Hot   ☐ Mild   ☐ Cold   BM Pressure: _____

☐ Dry   ☐ Humid   ☐ Wet   Allergen Levels: _____

☐ Sunny   ☐ Cloudy

STRESS LEVELS

None	Low	Medium	High	Max	@$#%!

FOOD / DRINKS + NON-RELIEF MEDICATION / SUPPLEMENTS

item / meal	time	meds / supplements	dose	time

How many drinks?

water → ① ② ③ ④ ⑤ ⑥ ⑦ ⑧ ⑨ ⑩

caffeine → ① ② ③ ④ ⑤ ⑥ ⑦ ⑧ ⑨ ⑩

alcohol → ① ② ③ ④ ⑤ ⑥ ⑦ ⑧ ⑨ ⑩

HORMONES

☐ Menstruating   ☐ Menopause   ☐ PMS   ☐ N/A | other

COMPUTER USE / READING

☐ None   ☐ Some   ☐ A lot   Total time: _____

☐ Sitting   ☐ Standing   ☐ Mixture   Breaks every: _____

PHYSICAL ACTIVITY

☐ None   ☐ Minimal   ☐ Some   ☐ Sweatin'   ☐ I'm beat

DETAILS: _____

RELIEF MEASURES

☐ Medication   ☐ Massage   ☐ Sleep   ☐ Exercise

☐ Water   ☐ Cold/Ice   ☐ Heat/Bath   ☐ Other

DETAILS: _____

DID IT WORK?   ☐ Nope   ☐ A bit   ☐ Mostly   ☐ 100%

Notes

Additional Notes